Tami A. Ross, RDN, LD, CDCES, MLDE, FAADE

WHAT DO I EAT NOW?

A Guide to Eating Well with Diabetes or Prediabetes

3rd Edition

Associate Publisher, Books, Abe Ogden*; Director, Book Operations,* Victor Van Beuren; *Managing Editor, Books,* John Clark; *Associate Director, Book Marketing,* Annette Reape; *Acquisitions Editor,* Jaclyn Konich; *Senior Manager, Book Editing,* Lauren Wilson; *Project Manager,* Wendy Martin-Shuma; *Composition,* Circle Graphics; *Cover Design,* Jenn French Designs; *Printer,* Versa Press.

Printed in the United States of America
1 3 5 7 9 10 8 6 4 2

The suggestions and information contained in this publication are generally consistent with the *Standards of Medical Care in Diabetes* and other policies of the American Diabetes Association, but they do not represent the policy or position of the Association or any of its boards or committees. Reasonable steps have been taken to ensure the accuracy of the information presented. However, the American Diabetes Association cannot ensure the safety or efficacy of any product or service described in this publication. Individuals are advised to consult a physician or other appropriate health care professional before undertaking any diet or exercise program or taking any medication referred to in this publication. Professionals must use and apply their own professional judgment, experience, and training and should not rely solely on the information contained in this publication before prescribing any diet, exercise, or medication. The American Diabetes Association—its officers, directors, employees, volunteers, and members—assumes no responsibility or liability for personal or other injury, loss, or damage that may result from the suggestions or information in this publication.

Shamera Robinson conducted the internal review of this book to ensure that it meets American Diabetes Association guidelines.

⊗ The paper in this publication meets the requirements of the ANSI Standard Z39.48-1992 (permanence of paper).

ADA titles may be purchased for business or promotional use or for special sales. To purchase more than 50 copies of this book at a discount, or for custom editions of this book with your logo, contact the American Diabetes Association at the address below or at booksales@diabetes.org.

American Diabetes Association
2451 Crystal Drive, Suite 900
Arlington, VA 22202

DOI: 10.2337/9781580407281

Library of Congress Cataloging-in-Publication Data

Names: Ross, Tami A., author.
Title: What do I eat now? : a guide to eating well with diabetes or
   prediabetes / Tami A. Ross, RDN, LD, CDCES, MLDE, FAADE.
Description: 3rd edition. | Arlington : American Diabetes Association,
   [2019] | Includes bibliographical references and index.
Identifiers: LCCN 2019038542 | ISBN 9781580407281 (paperback) | ISBN
   9781580407489 (ebook)
Subjects: LCSH: Diabetes—Diet therapy—Recipes. | Diabetics—Nutrition.
Classification: LCC RC662 .G452 2019 | DDC 641.5/6314—dc23
LC record available at https://lccn.loc.gov/2019038542

In memory of Patti Bazel Geil, my longtime friend, and coauthor
of the first and second editions of this book. Writing this third edition
without her was a challenge on many levels. I miss her every day.
–TAMI

TABLE OF CONTENTS

INTRODUCTION

What Do I Eat Now?

Perhaps you've just learned that you have type 2 diabetes or prediabetes. Or maybe you've had diabetes or prediabetes for some time and haven't been able to manage your blood glucose to the degree that you'd like. Whether you are newly diagnosed or have a newfound interest in self-care, you'll quickly discover that healthy eating is fundamental to taking good care of yourself and feeling your best. This book is designed for people with type 2 diabetes; however, the majority of the content and healthy eating tips can also be helpful for individuals managing prediabetes.

Undoubtedly, managing diabetes can feel like an overwhelming challenge at times. Research has shown that if an individual with type 2 diabetes who takes an oral medication followed all of the standard recommendations for self-care, **143 minutes of each day** would be spent on self-care tasks. That's almost 2 1/2 hours a day focused on diabetes care! Checking blood glucose, taking medication, exercising, and eating healthy may seem like a part-time job! It may not surprise you to find out that of those 143 minutes, almost half are related to food: planning, shopping, and preparing meals. Add to this the often-conflicting nutrition advice you may hear from others and the media. No wonder the biggest and most common question I hear is, "What do I eat now?"

Healthy Eating Should Be Pleasurable

Think about eating healthy as a journey. It is shaped by many factors, including what foods you like (and don't like), where you are in life, traditions and culture, and personal choices over time. Adopting a healthy eating pattern can help achieve the ultimate goal to improve overall health, including improving blood glucose, blood pressure, and blood lipid levels (i.e., cholesterol and triglycerides); achieving weight management goals; and delaying or preventing diabetes complications. The best plan is one that works for you to achieve your health goals, feel well, and live your best life. Food and eating are an important part of life. Eating should definitely be a pleasurable experience.

How This Book Can Help

Science and evidence are ever-evolving. All of the guidelines in this book are based on the latest scientific evidence at the time of publication. Throughout, I'll show you how to translate and use this information in everyday life to help fine-tune diabetes self-care and eating habits. Some steps may seem immediately manageable, while others may need more guidance. There is no "one size fits all" diet. You'll learn a variety of eating patterns, approaches, and tools to help. It's good to have options, because everyone is different. The end goal is finding what works for you to keep your blood glucose in range, and then doing more of that. As you read, you will see a multitude of practical illustrations and examples, many of which

I gleaned from clients over the course of my career. I hope you find them helpful, too!

Each chapter focuses on a different topic related to healthy eating with diabetes (or prediabetes). The content is broken down into sections, making it easy to jump around and focus on what you want to learn more about. At the end of each chapter, you will find Next Steps to take you toward healthy eating and Food for Thought, which contains a summary of information in the chapter.

Preparation Is the Secret to Success

The first step toward achieving success in embracing a healthy eating style for diabetes (or prediabetes) is to visualize what that success looks like for you.

What Are Your Health Goals?

- Eat healthier?
- Lose weight?
- Lower blood glucose?
- Feel better?
- Have more energy?
- Something else?

What Small Changes Come to Mind to Begin Building a Healthier Eating Style to Reach Your Health Goals?

- Will the foods you eat be different?
- Will the portions be different?
- Will your plate be portioned differently?
- Will you be making different choices in the grocery store and when dining out?

How Do You See Yourself Eating a Month from Now?

I challenge you to take the first step toward embracing a healthy eating style by imagining where you would like to be a month from now, and then start making plans to learn and do what you need to do to make your vision a reality.

Setting Goals and Taking Action

To help guide your plan, the first step is to set goals around eating, ideally for the next month. Depending on where you're at, you may decide to tackle just the next week, or the next day.

Are you familiar with SMART goals? SMART is an acronym for Specific, Measurable, Attainable, Relevant, and Timely. Your goal should have these five characteristics or qualities. SMART goal-setting gives you a framework for "getting it done." Using the SMART approach helps you reach your health goals, manage your time, and track your progress.

What Is a SMART Goal?

SPECIFIC: A specific goal has a greater chance of being achieved.

- What exactly do you want to accomplish? Answer who, what, when, where, how, and why.

MEASURABLE: Measuring progress keeps you on track.

- How can you track your progress? How will you know when you've reached your goal?

ATTAINABLE: An attainable goal is tied to small, easily accomplished steps.

- Is meeting this goal attainable or possible for you? If not, how will you get what you need to make it happen?

RELEVANT: A relevant goal is one you are willing and able to work toward.

- Why do you want to reach this goal? Is it important to you? Is it something you can do?

TIMELY: A deadline gives a sense of urgency and helps you to identify progress.

- When will you complete the goal? Set a time or deadline you can meet. Set a halfway measurement or milestone at which to check your progress.

3 Sample SMART Goals

1. **Initial goal:** I will eat more fruits and vegetables.
   SMART goal: I will have a medium fresh orange at lunch 3 days this week.
2. **Initial goal:** I will eat healthier when I'm on the road traveling for work several days a week.
   SMART goal: I will order a side salad instead of fries at lunch 2 days a week and have the dressing on the side so I can decide how much to put on the salad.
3. **Initial goal:** I will choose better snacks.
   SMART goal: I will eat a snack of almonds or pistachios that I portion out and bring from home instead of going to the vending machine every afternoon at work.

Give Your SMART Goal a "Stranger Test"

What do I mean by a "stranger test"? Make your goal specific enough that even if a stranger reads it, he or she will know what you plan to do.

Have an "If-Then" Statement for Your SMART Goal

Having an "if-then" statement ready provides options to help you achieve your goal if "life happens" and things do not go quite as planned. Here are a couple of examples of if-then statements:

- **SMART goal revolves around walking outside after work:** If it rains after work, then I'll walk on my treadmill instead.
- **SMART goal revolves around preparing healthy dinners at home:** If I get home late and can't prepare the meal I had planned, then I'll prepare a quick, healthy dinner from frozen items or pantry staples (such as foil-packed tuna, whole-grain crackers, and fruit).

Be Realistic

Sometimes life happens and you may not accomplish every goal you set, and that's okay. Do the best that you can. Having goals helps you maintain focus and keeps you moving onward and upward.

Behavior Is What You Do, Not What You Know

Diabetes is unlike other medical conditions in one key and unique way: *people with diabetes manage their own condition 95% of the time.*

There are seven key areas that require focus. These areas were identified by the Association of Diabetes Care and Education Specialists (formerly the AADE) and are known as the AADE7 Self-Care Behaviors:

1. Healthy Eating
2. Being Active
3. Monitoring
4. Taking Medication
5. Problem Solving
6. Reducing Risks
7. Healthy Coping

Healthy eating tops the list. It's not possible or practical to ask for medical advice every time you plan to eat, exercise, take medication, encounter an out-of-range blood glucose level, or deal with a minor illness. A diabetes care and education specialist can help you set priorities and coach you on each of these areas. A registered dietitian nutritionist (RDN) can provide personalized guidance on eating. Although you have a team of healthcare professionals, you are the one who will make the day-to-day decisions about your diabetes care.

Knowing what you need to do and actually *doing* it are two very different things. For instance, you may know that your diabetes healthcare team recommended you walk at least 30 minutes every day, but maybe you can't seem to find the time. Or maybe you know that your diabetes care and education specialist recommended you check your blood glucose at least twice each day, but sticking your finger is not fun, so you avoid it. And maybe you know that a third slice of pizza will send your blood glucose way out of range, but it just tastes so good. How many times have you said, "I know what I should do, but I just can't seem to do it"?

Stages of Change

Much research has been done in the area of behavior change. While working in the area of addiction, professor of psychology Dr. James Prochaska and colleagues developed the transtheoretical model of change as a way of explaining why certain individuals were able to change poor habits, while others were "stuck" and unable to adopt healthier actions. According to Prochaska's "stages of change" model, people are in different stages regarding their readiness to adopt a healthy behavior or stop an unhealthy one, and this affects their ability to change. These stages of change are:

- Pre-contemplation
- Contemplation
- Preparation
- Action
- Maintenance

Prochaska's work has been translated into the area of diabetes self-management education, helping health professionals match their education efforts and advice to the needs of the specific individual with diabetes at any one time, no matter which stage of change that individual currently occupies. Table 1 shows examples of how the stages of change might apply to someone with type 2 diabetes (or prediabetes) who is carrying a few extra pounds.

Although you may progress through the stages of change in an orderly fashion, change doesn't always come smoothly. At times, you may move one stage forward and then two stages back. But you can learn from what doesn't go well and then use that information to move forward again. For example, let's say you began a weight loss program at the first of the year, but because of stress at home and on the job, you've gone back to your old ways of eating and just can't find the energy to get back on track. Suddenly, you've moved from "action" back to "pre-contemplation." The important thing is to learn some healthy ways to cope with stress and move back into "action" again.

As you think about your life with diabetes, you may find that you're in a different stage of change for each area of the AADE7 Self-Care Behaviors. For example, you could be in the "maintenance" stage for Being Active because you've been walking 10,000 steps three times a week for the past year. However, you might still be in the "contemplation" stage regarding Monitoring because you are just beginning to realize the benefits that knowing your numbers (and responding) can have. Table 2 includes four of the AADE7 Self-Care Behaviors. Where are you in the stages of behavior change for each one?

TABLE 1   APPLYING THE STAGES OF CHANGE

Stage of Change	Characteristics	Weight Loss Example
Pre-contemplation	Unaware that change is needed or having no intention of changing.	"I feel fine, even though I might be a few pounds overweight."
Contemplation	Intends to change in the next 6 months; aware of the benefits and costs of change.	"I will try to lose some weight. It will help improve my blood glucose. But I don't know if I can give up my wife's good cooking."
Preparation	Ready to change in the next 30 days; taking steps to begin making a change.	"I've looked at all the diets out there. I think I'll stick with the eating plan the registered dietitian nutritionist made with me at my last visit."
Action	Has been making changes within the past 6 months.	"I've been following my meal plan and weighing myself every week for the past month."
Maintenance	Has successfully made a change for more than 6 months; making efforts to avoid slipping into past behaviors.	"Since the holidays are coming up, I need to plan on sticking with my current strategies, so I won't gain weight again this year."

TABLE 2   WHERE ARE YOU IN THE STAGES OF BEHAVIOR CHANGE?

Self-Care Behavior	Your Stage of Change
Healthy Eating	
Being Active (on a regular basis)	
Monitoring (your blood glucose)	
Taking Medications (if needed)	

A Goal Without a Plan Is Just a Wish

It's been said that a goal without a plan is just a wish. Take a moment to congratulate yourself on those behavior changes you may have already successfully accomplished. And for those areas that might still need work, I encourage you to consider setting SMART goals to help you continue to move forward. One of your goals could be to call on your diabetes healthcare team for additional guidance. Or you could schedule an appointment with an RDN to personalize what you learn in this book.

Prioritize the goals that are important to you. Which one will you work on first? Which will have the most impact on your health? List your goals in order of importance and then start with the first goal on the list. Taking these steps will focus your efforts, help you feel less overwhelmed, and reward you with a sense of accomplishment.

Consider the good things you're already doing, and do more of them or do them more often. Maybe you've switched from white bread to 100% whole-wheat bread. Or maybe you've been eating smaller portions at dinner. Keep doing that. I routinely hear from clients that over time, making those "better-for-you" food decisions soon becomes habit.

Eating healthy with diabetes is a journey, not a sprint. Eating healthy is shaped by many factors. All of your food and beverage choices count. If you commit to doing the best you can, then you've given it your best!

My hope is that when you finish this book, you will have the answer to "What do I eat now?" And that you will use this knowledge to help simplify life with diabetes and live the best life possible.

Next Steps

Set three SMART goals around healthy eating with diabetes. Keep the goals where you can look at them often. We'll revisit your goals in the last chapter. And celebrate positive changes you've put into action.

My SMART goals in priority order are:

1. _____

2. _____

3. _____

What are three changes you can make today to help you move toward accomplishing your #1 goal?

Food for Thought

- Healthy eating is shaped by many factors and should be pleasurable.
- The first step toward achieving success in embracing a healthy eating style for diabetes (or prediabetes) is to visualize what that success looks like for you.
- Setting SMART goals helps you reach your health goals, manage your time, and track your progress.
- Consider the good things you're already doing, and do more of them or do them more often.
- The road to healthy eating is a journey, not a sprint.

TYPE 2 DIABETES AND PREDIABETES: HOW THEY'RE RELATED AND WHAT YOU NEED TO KNOW

Millions of people around the world live with diabetes, or know someone who does. The majority of people who have diabetes have what's known as *type 2 diabetes*. However, even more common is *prediabetes*. Before we dive in and answer the question, "What do I eat now?," I want to make sure we start on the same page with a brief review of the basics you need to know about type 2 diabetes and prediabetes, and how they are related.

Diabetes Defined

Diabetes is a chronic condition where blood glucose builds up in the blood (also known as "blood sugar"), leading to levels higher than normal, which can cause problems if not managed.

There are three main forms of diabetes:

- **Type 2 diabetes:** This is the most common form of diabetes. Although once called "adult-onset diabetes," type 2 diabetes can actually occur at any age. If you have type 2 diabetes, your body does not use insulin properly, and this condition is called "insulin resistance." Insulin's job is to help keep the right amount of glucose (sugar) in your blood to fuel your body. When someone has insulin resistance, the fat, liver, and muscle cells do not respond normally to insulin, and, as a result, the pancreas produces more and more insulin. Over time, the pancreas isn't able to keep up with the increased need, and blood glucose levels rise above normal.

- **Type 1 diabetes:** Previously known as "juvenile" diabetes, type 1 diabetes can actually occur at any age as well (and in people of every race, shape, and size). In fact, there are currently more adults than children with type 1 diabetes. In people with type 1 diabetes, the body stops making insulin altogether, so the individual must take life-saving insulin to live.
- **Gestational diabetes:** Gestational diabetes is high blood glucose that is first identified during pregnancy after the first trimester. Gestational diabetes is also tied to insulin resistance. Hormones from the placenta, which supports the baby as it grows, block insulin action. The pregnant woman may need much more insulin as a result to "overcome" the resistance. If her body can't produce enough, blood glucose levels rise above normal. Women who have had gestational diabetes should have lifelong screening for type 2 diabetes or prediabetes at least every 3 years.

Prediabetes: Stepping Toward Type 2 Diabetes

Prediabetes occurs when blood glucose levels are slightly higher than normal, but not high enough to fall into the diabetes range. As the name implies, prediabetes comes before type 2 diabetes. *Having prediabetes is basically the first step toward type 2 diabetes.* Many people with

prediabetes go on to develop type 2 diabetes within 10 years. Current estimates from the Centers for Disease Control and Prevention (CDC) are that one in three American adults has prediabetes. And most are unaware of the condition.

Think about prediabetes this way: it is like a yellow caution light. Being diagnosed with prediabetes is a warning that type 2 diabetes may be ahead. There are often no symptoms with prediabetes. However, prediabetes can still cause problems and lead to increased risk for heart disease and stroke. The really positive news is this: *prediabetes responds well to healthy eating habits, weight loss, and exercise—what may also be known as "lifestyle change."* We focus more on lifestyle change later in this chapter.

How Prediabetes and Diabetes Are Diagnosed: What the Numbers Mean

Here are a few explanations about the lab tests and values the healthcare team uses to diagnose prediabetes or diabetes:

- **Fasting blood glucose level** is taken when you've had nothing to eat or drink, except water, for 8 hours before the test.
- **2-hour oral glucose tolerance test** is a special test during which you are given a sweet drink that contains a specific amount of glucose (a sugar), and your blood glucose levels are checked 2 hours later.

TABLE 1.1   BLOOD GLUCOSE LEVELS USED TO DIAGNOSE PREDIABETES AND DIABETES

Diagnosis	Fasting Blood Glucose Level	2-Hour Glucose Level on Oral Glucose Tolerance Test	A1C (%)
Normal blood glucose	<100	<140 mg/dL	<5.7
Prediabetes	100–125 mg/dL	140–199 mg/dL	5.7–6.4
Diabetes	≥126 mg/dL	≥200 mg/dL	≥6.5

- A1C provides an estimation of average blood glucose over the past 2–3 months and doesn't require fasting or a glucose drink.
- A **random blood glucose test** can be taken at any time of day to diagnose diabetes. This test is often used when a person shows classic diabetes symptoms (these symptoms are discussed later in the chapter). Diabetes is diagnosed when a random blood glucose level is ≥200 mg/dL and the patient has classic symptoms of hyperglycemia or a hyperglycemic crisis. See Table 1.1 for glucose levels that diagnose diabetes and prediabetes.

The Path to Type 2 Diabetes

Normal blood glucose: <100 mg/dL

↓

Prediabetes: 100–125 mg/dL

↓

Type 2 diabetes: ≥126 mg/dL

Symptoms of High Blood Glucose

Type 2 diabetes usually develops gradually, and its symptoms can be so subtle that they may go unnoticed for a while. The symptoms that follow occur as a result of glucose (sugar) building up in the blood. Looking back, you might realize that you had some of the classic diabetes symptoms even before you were diagnosed. The symptoms may include:

- Feeling extra thirsty
- Urinating more often
- Unusual tiredness and fatigue
- Feeling very hungry
- Blurry vision
- Cuts and bruises that are slow to heal
- Unexplained weight loss
- Tingling, pain, or numbness in your hands or feet
- Dry or itchy skin
- Recurring infections

Many people ignore these symptoms or simply chalk them up to "getting older." They may put off visiting their healthcare provider because the symptoms don't seem serious, which further delays the diabetes diagnosis.

If you have already been diagnosed with type 2 diabetes, your family members may be at increased risk for the condition. Diabetes tends to run in families. It may be helpful to know that the healthy eating guidance you'll learn from this book can be helpful for the whole family to embrace, to delay or prevent type 2 diabetes. Healthy eating patterns can also provide benefits with respect to blood pressure, body weight, and lipid profiles.

Blood Glucose Goals and Why They Matter

Diabetes can be managed. Evidence shows that keeping your blood glucose as close to normal as possible without experiencing frequent low blood glucose can help prevent long-term complications associated with diabetes (such as damage to the heart, eyes, feet, kidneys, and nerves). Managing blood pressure and blood lipids (total cholesterol, LDL cholesterol, and triglycerides) is also important to help prevent future problems.

Table 1.2 presents the general goals recommended by the American Diabetes Association. These goals are provided as a point of reference. *It's important to talk with your healthcare team about what the best goals are for you.*

How Is Food Related to Rising Blood Glucose Levels?

To put it simply, when you eat food or drink beverages that have carbohydrate, your body breaks down the carbohydrate into a sugar called glucose (see Chapter 4 for more on

TABLE 1.2   GOALS FROM THE AMERICAN DIABETES ASSOCIATION
Blood glucose   • Preprandial (before eating): 80–130 mg/dL   • Peak postprandial (after eating): <180 mg/dL (when blood glucose is generally peaking 1–2 hours after beginning a meal)   • A1C <7.0%
Blood pressure   • <140/90 mmHg for individuals at higher risk for heart disease   • <130/80 mmHg for individuals at lower risk for heart disease
Blood lipids   • LDL ("bad") cholesterol: Targets vary when factoring in cardiovascular risk. Lower is better. Consult with your healthcare team. Statins are the drugs of choice for lowering LDL cholesterol.   • HDL ("good") cholesterol: >40 mg/dL in men or >50 mg/dL in women   • Triglycerides: <150 mg/dL

carbohydrates). Glucose is then absorbed into the bloodstream, where it is called "blood glucose" (or "blood sugar"). This glucose is then escorted out of the blood by insulin (a hormone made by your pancreas) into the body's cells, where it is used to fuel your body. With prediabetes or type 2 diabetes, either insulin isn't working well to move glucose out of the blood, or your body stops making enough insulin to do the job.

Other Factors That Affect Blood Glucose

There are actually over 40 identified factors that can affect blood glucose. You'll learn much more about the food-related factors throughout this book. Other factors that broadly affect blood glucose levels include the following:

- **Physical activity** (including type of activity, fitness level, time of day, and food and medication timing)
- **Medication** if any (dose, timing, interactions, and type)
- **Biological factors** (including sleep, stress, illness, hypoglycemia, blood glucose overnight, allergies, menstruation, and tobacco use)
- **Environmental factors** (including temperature, sunburn, and altitude)
- **Behavior/decision-making** (including issues with family relationships and social pressures)

There are many ways to make small changes to help affect and manage blood glucose.

The diaTribe website (www.diatribe.org) addresses these many factors. diaTribe is a patient-focused online publication that helps The diaTribe Foundation to carry out its mission to improve the lives of people with diabetes.

Type 2 Diabetes Is a Progressive Condition

A progressive condition is one in which the body's insulin-producing cells gradually lose their ability to function well over time. It does not mean, though, that your diabetes is getting "worse." Don't blame yourself. *Would you blame yourself if you needed stronger glasses because your eyesight changed?* Treatments such as oral medications, injectable medications, or both may be needed—in addition to healthy eating, physical activity, and behavior change—to manage blood glucose. If your healthcare team recommends starting, changing, or adding a medication (or two or three medications) to help manage blood glucose, it does not mean your best efforts at healthy eating and lifestyle change have failed. Healthy eating continues to be a core part of diabetes management across your lifetime. As time goes on, it, too, may need tweaks.

Can Type 2 Diabetes Be Prevented?

When looking back on blood glucose over time, many notice levels gradually creeping up each year on lab work. Recognizing this developing condition, especially as blood glucose hits the prediabetes range, and taking action, can help hold off or prevent going on to develop type 2 diabetes. Substantial evidence has shown the following three lifestyle changes can significantly reduce the incidence of going on to develop type 2 diabetes:

- **Lifestyle Change #1:** Improve eating habits and food quality.
- **Lifestyle Change #2:** Get moderate-intensity physical activity at least 150 minutes per week.
- **Lifestyle Change #3:** Maintain a 7–10% weight loss (if overweight).

You'll learn more about lifestyle change in Chapter 2. The impact of these lifestyle changes was noted in a large research study called the Diabetes Prevention Program. These changes helped reduce the chance of prediabetes developing into type 2 diabetes by 58%. In addition to the lifestyle changes, some healthcare professionals may recommend a medication called metformin to help prevent type 2 diabetes. Metformin is also prescribed to help manage type 2 diabetes. It is inexpensive, effective, and does not cause weight gain. In fact, many notice modest weight loss when taking metformin. So if your healthcare team recommends metformin, it does not mean things are "in really bad shape." Starting this medication is just another option to help hold off type 2 diabetes. If you have prediabetes, I encourage you to join a Diabetes Prevention Program in your

area (also known as DPP). Find a DPP near you at https://nccd.cdc.gov/DDT_DPRP/ Registry.aspx. This program is built on the lifestyle changes that were found effective in the DPP study. Health insurance plans often cover the DPP for individuals at risk for developing type 2 diabetes.

Let's review more about the three lifestyle changes to help prevent diabetes. (These changes are also beneficial in managing type 2 diabetes, and we'll talk more about them in the next chapter). Every small change you are able to make can help. Small changes can really add up.

Lifestyle Change #1: Improve Eating Habits and Food Quality

What you eat has a big impact on your blood glucose levels. Making healthy choices in what you eat and drink can help manage blood glucose. Overall, the goal is to build your eating around nutrient-dense foods. That means eating foods that are rich in vitamins, minerals, and fiber—foods that are less processed and closer to nature (instead of foods laden with added fat, sugar, or sodium). These high-quality foods include vegetables, fruits, beans, legumes, pulses, low-fat milk and dairy, lean protein, nuts, seeds, and whole grains.

If you have prediabetes and are at a healthy weight, a Mediterranean-style eating pattern can be beneficial. You may have heard of the Mediterranean way of eating. You'll learn much more about how to eat Mediterranean-style in Chapter 2.

4 Swaps to Make the Move Toward Higher-Quality Food Throughout the Day

1. **At breakfast:** Rather than eating a processed cereal, work in a whole grain by swapping in oats. Don't like mushy quick oats? Then try steel-cut oats. They take longer to cook, so cook a larger batch and freeze in muffin tins for a perfectly portioned ready-to-microwave breakfast.

2. **At lunch:** Rather than chips or pretzels, swap in carrots for crunch.

3. **At dinner:** Rather than white rice, swap in quinoa, a whole grain. Or expand your horizons with nutty-tasting millet or farro. There are frozen and microwavable forms to keep dinner prep simple.

4. **At snacks:** Rather than a cookie or other sweet treat, grab a small piece of fruit that doesn't need to be prepped. Start with a clementine or plum, for instance.

Lifestyle Change #2: Get Moderate-Intensity Physical Activity at Least 150 Minutes Per Week

Regular physical activity is beneficial not only for preventing type 2 diabetes, but also for managing type 2 diabetes.

Structured Physical Activity (Exercise) Has a Number of Positive Effects

- Lowers blood glucose during and after activity
- Strengthens the heart muscle, which lowers blood pressure and resting heart rate
- Reduces total cholesterol and triglycerides and increases HDL cholesterol (the "good" cholesterol)
- Assists with weight loss and management by regulating appetite and boosting calorie burning
- Aids in stress management and improves well-being, which in turn may lead to lower blood glucose levels

What Counts as Moderate-Intensity Physical Activity?

Examples of moderate-intensity aerobic activities include the following:

- Brisk walking (walking a mile in 17 minutes)
- Cycling
- Dancing
- Swimming
- Tennis (doubles)
- Gardening

The goal is to raise your heart rate, which is the number of times your heart beats per minute. With moderate-intensity physical activity, your heart beats at 50–70% of your maximum heart rate. According to the American Heart Association, your maximum heart rate is about 220 minus your age.

> ## Let's Do the Math
>
> If you're 60 years old, your maximum heart rate is about 160 beats per minute (220 – 60 = 160); 50–70% of that maximum heart rate is about 80–112 beats per minute. That would be your target heart rate when exercising.

Try to Reduce Sedentary Time

Prolonged sitting is harmful to health. The recommendation from health authorities, which is loud and clear, is to decrease the amount of time spent in sedentary activity (such as desk work, watching TV, or playing videogames). The goal for adults is to get up every 30 minutes and stand briefly (around 5 minutes) or engage in 3 minutes of light walking and simple body weight resistance activities (such as lunges, pushups against the wall, or sit and stand). These activity breaks benefit blood glucose.

Lifestyle Change #3: Maintain a 7–10% Weight Loss (If Overweight)

Again, there is strong evidence clearly showing that modest weight loss (and keeping it off) can delay progression from prediabetes to type 2 diabetes, and this weight loss is also helpful in managing type 2 diabetes. Weight loss helps lower morning fasting glucose (before you eat or drink anything), which is important when trying to manage prediabetes and type 2 diabetes. Experiencing above-normal fasting glucose can be a challenge for people with prediabetes or type 2 diabetes.

> ## Let's Do the Math
>
> For someone who's 200 pounds, losing 7% of their body weight would translate into losing 14 pounds. Losing 10% would translate into losing 20 pounds. Many find these goals doable.

Set Mini–Weight Loss Milestones

I encourage you to set mini–weight loss milestones. Celebrate every 5 pounds you lose! By setting mini-goals, you increase your chances of an early victory, with the small wins serving as motivators to bigger wins down the road.

Energy Balance Is Important in Delaying or Preventing Type 2 Diabetes

Balancing energy intake (calories from food and beverages) with energy expenditure (calories burnt off through physical activity) leads to weight maintenance. To achieve weight loss means altering that balance—burning off more calories than you eat or drink.

The amount of calories you need is based on a number of things, including your age, gender, height, weight, and physical activity.

- **Generally, trimming 500–750 calories off each day can lead to weight loss.**
- **Women can often lose weight by reducing calories to around 1,200–1,500 per day.**

- **Men can often lose weight by reducing calories to around 1,500–1,800 per day.**

Ask Yourself: "Are the Calories Worth It?"

For instance, a 150-pound woman would have to dance energetically for about 40 minutes to burn off the calories in a slice of apple pie. Or she would have to cycle about 10 minutes

---

Small Changes Cut Calories

Small changes cut calories and add up. Make all of the small swaps below and save over 1,000 calories!

- **Drink water or another zero-calorie beverage** instead of a regular soda, sweet tea, lemonade, or juice drink. This change saves about 250 calories for each 20-ounce drink swap.
- **Go for foods that aren't fried.** The calorie and fat savings can be dramatic. Enjoy 5 ounces of grilled fished instead of fried fish, and save 234 calories.
- **Use reduced-fat (light) or fat-free versions** of high-fat foods, such as sour cream, cream cheese, mayonnaise, cheese, and salad dressing. Use buttery spray on vegetables instead of margarine or butter, and save 65 calories per tablespoon. Replace mayonnaise with creamy Dijon mustard, and save 75 calories per tablespoon.
- **Swap in whole grains.** Substitute whole-wheat pasta, brown rice, and whole-wheat bread for the more refined white versions. The fiber will help you feel full, so you will likely be satisfied with smaller portions.
- **Chew, don't drink.** Enjoy a crunchy 4-ounce apple instead of 12 ounces of natural apple juice, and save 122 calories. Plus you get the sensory benefit from chewing.
- **Swap in nonstarchy vegetables.** Pump up the flavor in an omelet with 1/4 cup pepper and onions instead of 1/4 cup shredded cheese to save 200 calories. Swap in mashed cauliflower for mashed potatoes, and save 100 calories per cup. A list of nonstarchy vegetable options can be found on page 50.

to burn off the calories in a 1-ounce cube of cheese.

Save Calories with Small Switches

Switch a 20-ounce sweet tea or cola to water or other zero-calorie beverage and save 250 calories. Do that twice a day, and you've trimmed 500 calories. Do that every day for a week, and you've trimmed 3,500 calories. That one change can lead to weight loss!

Meet with a Registered Dietitian Nutritionist (RDN)

I encourage you to meet with a registered dietitian nutritionist (RDN) for personalized guidance on a calorie level that is best for you, along with guidance on how to incorporate high-quality foods into your eating pattern. Until then, you may find a free calorie-tracker app helpful. There are many out there. Favorites among my clients have been MyFitnessPal, Lose It!, and MyPlate Calorie Counter.

The goal is to find something you can do and stick with long term. Sustaining weight loss, while challenging, does have long-term benefits. Maintaining weight loss for 5 years is associated with sustained improvements in A1C and lipid levels.

What Are Your Goals for Diabetes Management?

You won't learn everything you need to know about managing diabetes just by reading this book or going to one appointment with an RDN or diabetes care and education specialist. It's vitally important that you and your diabetes healthcare team discuss your personal goals for blood glucose, blood pressure, and blood lipids. Your goals for living well with diabetes (or prediabetes) may differ from the American Diabetes Association recommendations shared earlier in the chapter. Or they may be different than recommendations of other family members, friends, or acquaintances with diabetes.

Next Steps

1. Reflect on changes you may have already made. What is going well now?
2. How can you do more of what is going well to continue down the path toward living your best life?
3. Assess your physical activity. Do you get 150 minutes each week? If not, identify where in your day and how can you fit in more fitness.
4. Could you benefit from dropping a few pounds? If so, what is one swap you can make to cut calories?

Food for Thought

- Prediabetes is the first step toward type 2 diabetes. With lifestyle change, there is over a 50% chance you can delay or halt the progression.
- Prediabetes and type 2 diabetes respond well to weight loss, healthy eating, and regular physical activity.
- Type 2 diabetes is a progressive condition. Healthy eating, physical activity, and behavior change are the foundation for diabetes management, but new medications and therapies may need to be added over time.

HOW LIFESTYLE CHANGES HELP

Lifestyle change—we hear that term used frequently. *But what does it mean?* Think about lifestyle change as a positive change process to become different—to become a different you. Lifestyle change is a process that begins with small steps, small swaps, and small changes in what you eat, how you manage weight, how you move, and how you manage stress. This book focuses primarily on the "what to eat" piece of lifestyle to help you live your best life, but keep in mind that healthy eating does not stand alone.

Changing lifestyle is a journey, not a sprint. (And that journey may be bumpy at times because "life happens.") Changing lifestyle takes time and support. Once you are ready to change (that means you are in the Preparation stage of change, discussed in the Introduction), it's time for careful planning and taking things one step at a time. In Chapter 1, you learned about how lifestyle, particularly weight loss and physical activity, affects blood glucose. This chapter builds on that information with additional practical and doable guidance. Small changes add up and make a difference. Lifestyle is a core influencer on diabetes care.

Healthy Eating: A Special Focus on Type 2 Diabetes

Nutrition has long been recognized as the cornerstone of successful diabetes management. Without a doubt, what you eat has a big impact on your blood glucose levels. Even as far back as 1550 B.C., doctors in some parts of the world recommended that people with diabetes follow a diet of wheat grain, fresh grits, grapes, honey berries, and sweet beer to replace the sugar lost through the urine. Today's recommendations are quite different! Making healthy choices in what you eat and drink can help manage blood glucose. The following is a summary of the overarching goals of eating well with diabetes.

Goals for Eating Well with Diabetes

- **Embrace a healthful eating pattern that includes a variety of nutrient-dense foods, and manage portions to improve overall health and reach blood glucose, blood pressure, and lipid goals.** A variety of healthy eating patterns for diabetes will be discussed in Chapter 3. Nutrient-rich foods are those that are rich in vitamins, minerals, and fiber—foods that are less processed and closer to nature (as opposed to foods laden with added fat, sugar, or sodium). If you don't know what blood glucose, blood pressure, and lipid goals are right for you, ask your diabetes healthcare team. Refer back to page 4 in Chapter 1 for a review of the general goals for blood glucose, blood pressure, and blood lipids from the American Diabetes Association.
- **Achieve and maintain body weight goals.** You'll learn more on this topic later in this chapter.
- **Delay or prevent complications of diabetes.** Refer back to Chapter 1 on page 4 for ways to delay diabetes complications.

- **Factor in individual nutrition needs.** These needs include personal and cultural preferences, access to healthful food choices, willingness and ability to make changes, and any barriers to change.
- **Maintain the pleasure of eating. Limit foods only when necessary to achieve your health goals.** For instance, if you have high blood pressure, scientific evidence shows that reducing salt (sodium) and salty foods can help lower blood pressure, so salt (sodium) reduction may help you achieve your health goals. (Reducing sodium lower than 2,300 mg/day should be considered only on an individual basis.)
- **Taking a practical approach is important,** rather than focusing on individual nutrients or single foods.

Dietary Guidelines for Americans: The Foundation of Eating Healthy

The quest to eat more healthfully begins with having a solid foundation, and the *Dietary Guidelines for Americans 2015–2020* (DGA) provides that. The DGA is updated approximately every 5 years based on new findings. These guidelines provide broad guidance and a foundation for healthy eating for *all* Americans. You can find these guidelines online if you wish to review the entire publication (visit https://health.gov/dietaryguidelines/2015/resources/2015-2020_Dietary_Guidelines.pdf).

Basically, the DGA stresses the importance of finding and creating a healthy way of eating (called a *healthy eating pattern*) and building on that behavior throughout life to keep you healthier now and in the future. Here is a summary of the basic guidelines.

According to the DGA, a healthy eating pattern includes the following:

- A variety of vegetables
- Fruits
- Grains
- Lower-fat dairy
- A variety of protein foods
- Oils

A healthy eating pattern limits the following:

- Saturated fats
- Trans fats
- Added sugars
- Sodium

Are You Eating Healthy?

To help you begin to get in touch with how your eating habits measure up to the DGA, answer the following questions. Any questions that you answer as "no" or "sometimes" can identify opportunities for positive change. You'll learn more about each of these as you make your way through the book.

- Do you eat a variety of vegetables?
- Do you eat vegetables and/or fruit at most meals?
- Do you eat at least 1 1/2 cups of vegetables a day?
- Do you eat more nonstarchy vegetables than the starchy variety? (See listing in Chapter 3 on page 50.)
- Do you eat 1 cup of fruit a day?
- Do you choose whole fruit more often than fruit juice?
- Do you eat at least three small servings of whole grains each day?
- Do you use lower-fat dairy (skim, 1%, or 2% milk; reduced-fat or fat-free cheese)?
- Do you eat protein-rich foods like fish, poultry, meat, soy foods, or eggs at most meals?
- Do you eat naturally fatty fish like tuna, salmon, lake trout, and herring at least twice a week?
- Do you limit solid fats, animal fats, and fatty cuts of meat?
- Do you use liquid oils like olive oil more often than butter and solid spreads?
- Do you avoid sugary drinks like regular soda, sweet tea, fruit punch, and regular lemonade?
- Do you choose foods naturally low in sodium or lower-sodium versions?

Again, the DGA gives perspective and a place to start as you move toward eating healthy. As you make your way through the book, you will learn much more about each of the foods and nutrients to include, as well as those to limit. You'll also learn about specific modifications in the types of foods you select and portions to help manage blood glucose. Small changes can help build a healthier eating style.

3 Small Changes Toward a Healthier Eating Style

1. **Brighten up your plate with vegetables that are red, orange, yellow, and dark green.** The different colors provide different nutrients.
2. **Choose whole fruit instead of juice.** Whole fruit has more fiber, is more satisfying, and will not raise blood glucose as quickly as juice.
3. **Choose bread, crackers, or cereals that are whole grain.** Look for the words "100% whole wheat" or "100% whole grain" on the label. The goal is that at least half the grains you eat are whole grains. Whole grains have more fiber and nutrients than processed grains.

MyPlate: An Illustration of Healthy Eating

To illustrate the DGA in a way that is understandable and doable at a glance, MyPlate was created. Most people have heard the phrase "a picture is worth a thousand words." MyPlate illustrates what a healthy meal looks like based on the DGA. If you're not familiar with MyPlate, here's what it looks like.

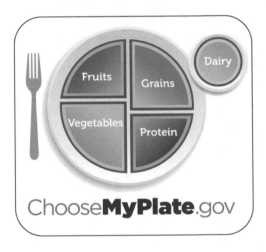

MyPlate serves as a reminder to find your healthy eating style and build on it throughout your lifetime. Everything you eat and drink matters. MyPlate is general guidance provided for reference, to give you perspective and get you focused on a healthy meal makeup. *However, MyPlate is portioned with too much carbohydrate for most people with diabetes. You will learn more about carbohydrate in the next few chapters. And, in Chapter 3, you'll learn how to make a few adjustments to portion your plate to better suit your needs for managing blood glucose.*

8 Tips to Guide You in the Quest to Find Your Healthy Eating Style and Maintain It for a Lifetime

1. Know that everything you eat and drink day-to-day throughout your life matters. The right mix can help keep you be healthier now and in the future.
2. Focus on including a variety of foods and colors at each meal to get a variety of flavors and nutrients.
3. Adjust portions to help manage weight and blood glucose. You'll learn how to do this in Chapter 7.
4. Start with small changes or swaps to build a healthier eating style, instead of going for a total overhaul from the start, which may feel overwhelming.
5. Take it one meal, one day at a time. Healthy eating doesn't mean always being perfect. There will be days when things go as planned and days that they just don't for any number of reasons.
6. The foods that are good for you are good for everyone in the family.
7. Team up with someone to help you stay on track, whether it's a friend, family member, your healthcare team, online support, or another form of support.
8. Celebrate each positive change or success as you build healthy eating habits.

Eating Healthy Is a Journey

Eating healthy is a journey shaped by many factors, as mentioned earlier in this chapter under Goals for Eating Well with Diabetes. Your stage of life, situation, preferences, access to food, culture, traditions, and the personal decisions you make over time all are important to consider. All your food and beverage choices count on this journey.

Now that you know the foundation to healthy eating, we'll begin to build and expand on that throughout the rest of the book. Hopefully, you are thinking about small changes or swaps you can begin to make to build a stronger foundation as you make positive changes in your lifestyle. Let's turn now and focus on another lifestyle area that has a big impact on diabetes—how you manage your weight.

Weighty Issues

The vast majority of individuals with type 2 diabetes are overweight and have insulin resistance. Many also have high blood pressure and high blood lipids. Weight loss is an important part of therapy for improving all aspects of type 2 diabetes. In Chapter 1, we discussed that maintaining a 7–10% weight loss (if overweight) can help *delay or prevent* type 2 diabetes. Weight management is not only critical for preventing type 2 diabetes, but also for *managing* type 2 diabetes. Losing at least 5% of your body weight helps lower not only blood glucose, but also blood pressure and lipids. Weight loss benefits are progressive. *More intensive goals, such as losing 15% or more of your body weight,* when feasible and can be safely accomplished, are associated with even better outcomes. Basically, the thing to know is weight loss helps, and generally, the greater the weight loss, the greater the benefits. Small changes can yield big results.

Let's Do the Math

For people who are 200 pounds, losing 5% of their weight would translate into losing 10 pounds. Many find that doable.

For people who are 150 pounds, losing 5% of their weight would translate into losing 7 1/2 pounds. Again, many find that doable.

How Do You Know If You Are at a Healthy Weight?

If your weight is a concern, you can start managing it by determining your weight status. A measurement known as the body mass index (BMI) takes into account your height and weight, making BMI a reliable indicator of body fat (Table 2.1 and 2.2). Your healthcare team may calculate your BMI at your visits. If you aren't familiar with your BMI, there are several ways you can determine this measurement:

- **Refer to an online BMI chart.** Locate your height in the left column and read across the row for that height to find your weight. Follow the column of the weight up to the top row, which lists your BMI.
- **Use an online BMI calculator.** There are many. You can find one at the website for the National Heart, Lung, and Blood Institute (https://www.nhlbi.nih.gov/health/educational/lose_wt/BMI/bmicalc.htm).
- **Calculate it yourself.** Multiply your height in inches times your height in inches. Then, divide your weight in pounds by that number. Finally, multiply that result by 703. That's your BMI.

Let's Do the Math

For someone 5'5" (65 inches) tall and weighing 180 pounds:

- Multiply height in inches × height in inches: $65 \times 65 = 4{,}225$
- Divide weight in pounds by that number: 180 divided by 4,225 = 0.04260355
- Multiply that by 703: $0.04260355 \times 703 = 29.95$, which rounds up to 30
- BMI = 30 kg/m^2

TABLE 2.1   BMI CHART

BMI (kg/m²)	Normal						Overweight					Obese					
	19	20	21	22	23	24	25	26	27	28	29	30	31	32	33	34	35
Height (inches)	Body Weight (pounds)																
58	91	96	100	105	110	115	119	124	129	134	138	143	148	153	158	162	167
59	94	99	104	109	114	119	124	128	133	138	143	148	153	158	163	168	173
60	97	102	107	112	118	123	128	133	138	143	148	153	158	163	168	174	179
61	100	106	111	116	122	127	132	137	143	148	153	158	164	169	174	180	185
62	104	109	115	120	126	131	136	142	147	153	158	164	169	175	180	186	191
63	107	113	118	124	130	135	141	146	152	158	163	169	175	180	186	191	197
64	110	116	122	128	134	140	145	151	157	163	169	174	180	186	192	197	204
65	114	120	126	132	138	144	150	156	162	168	174	180	186	192	198	204	210
66	118	124	130	136	142	148	155	161	167	173	179	186	192	198	204	210	216
67	121	127	134	140	146	153	159	166	172	178	185	191	198	204	211	217	223
68	125	131	138	144	151	158	164	171	177	184	190	197	203	210	216	223	230
69	128	135	142	149	155	162	169	176	182	189	196	203	209	216	223	230	236
70	132	139	146	153	160	167	174	181	188	195	202	209	216	222	229	236	243
71	136	143	150	157	165	172	179	186	193	200	208	215	222	229	236	243	250
72	140	147	154	162	169	177	184	191	199	206	213	221	228	235	242	250	258
73	144	151	159	166	174	182	189	197	204	212	219	227	235	242	250	257	265
74	148	155	163	171	179	186	194	202	210	218	225	233	241	249	256	264	272
75	152	160	168	176	184	192	200	208	216	224	232	240	248	256	164	272	279
76	156	164	172	180	189	197	205	213	221	230	238	246	254	263	271	279	287

(continued)

TABLE 2.1   BMI CHART (Continued)

BMI (kg/m²)	Extreme obesity																		
	36	37	38	39	40	41	42	43	44	45	46	47	48	49	50	51	52	53	54
Height (inches)	Body Weight (pounds)																		
58	172	177	181	186	191	196	201	205	210	215	220	224	229	234	239	244	248	253	258
59	178	183	188	193	198	203	208	212	217	222	227	232	237	242	247	252	257	262	267
60	184	189	194	199	204	209	215	22	225	230	235	240	245	250	255	261	266	271	276
61	190	195	201	206	211	217	222	227	232	238	243	248	254	259	264	269	275	280	285
62	196	202	207	213	218	224	229	235	240	246	251	256	262	267	273	278	284	289	295
63	203	208	214	220	225	231	237	242	248	254	259	265	270	278	282	287	293	299	304
64	209	215	221	227	232	238	244	250	256	262	267	273	279	285	291	296	301	308	314
65	216	222	228	234	240	246	252	258	264	270	276	282	288	294	300	306	312	318	324
66	223	229	235	241	247	253	260	266	272	278	284	291	297	303	309	315	322	328	334
67	230	236	242	149	255	261	268	274	280	287	293	299	306	312	319	325	331	338	344
68	236	243	249	256	262	269	276	282	289	295	302	308	315	322	328	335	341	348	354
69	243	250	257	263	270	277	284	291	297	304	311	318	324	331	338	345	351	358	365
70	250	257	264	271	278	285	292	299	306	313	320	327	334	341	348	355	362	369	376
71	257	265	272	279	286	293	301	308	315	322	329	338	343	351	358	365	372	379	386
72	265	272	279	287	294	302	309	316	324	331	338	346	353	361	368	375	383	390	397
73	272	280	288	295	302	310	318	325	333	340	348	355	363	371	378	386	393	401	408
74	280	287	295	303	311	319	326	334	342	350	358	365	373	381	389	396	404	412	420
75	287	295	303	311	319	327	335	343	351	359	367	375	383	391	399	407	415	423	431
76	295	304	312	320	328	336	344	353	361	369	377	385	394	402	410	418	426	435	443

National Heart, Lung, and Blood Institute. Body mass index table. Available from https://www.nhlbi.nih.gov/health/educational/lose_wt/BMI/bmi_tbl.htm.

TABLE 2.2 ARE YOU OVERWEIGHT, UNDERWEIGHT, OR JUST RIGHT? USE YOUR BMI TO FIND OUT	
BMI (kg/m²)	**Weight Status**
<18.5	Underweight
18.5–24.9	Normal weight
25.0–29.9	Overweight*
≥30	Obese

*Recent findings note that Asian Americans are at an increased risk for diabetes at lower BMI levels relative to the general population. "Overweight" for Asian Americans is a BMI of 23 kg/m².

As body fat or BMI increases above the ideal, health risks also increase. Being overweight (BMI of 25–29.9 kg/m²) or being obese (BMI ≥30 kg/m²) increases the risk of having high blood pressure, heart disease, stroke, diabetes, certain types of cancer, arthritis, and breathing problems. Research shows that being obese lowers your life expectancy.

How to Get Started Working Toward a Healthier Weight

If you discovered that you can stand to drop a few pounds, here are three tips to jumpstart your progress.

Tip #1: Balance Your Calories

You learned in Chapter 1 that energy balance is important to delay and prevent type 2 diabetes, but balancing energy also plays an important role in managing type 2 diabetes. Burning off more calories than you eat or drink can help you lose weight. Enhancing physical activity can help with that.

- **Generally, trimming 500–750 calories off each day can lead to weight loss.**
- **Women can often lose weight by reducing calories to around 1,200–1,500 per day.**
- **Men can often lose weight by reducing calories to around 1,500–1,800 per day.**

Save Calories with Small Switches

Swap fish for steak: Swap a 3-ounce serving of grilled whitefish (80 calories) in place of a 3-ounce serving of grilled ribeye steak (225 calories). That switch saves 145 calories. Make this change once a week and you'll cut over 7,500 calories in a year! That is enough calorie savings to lose about 2 pounds.

Swap avocado for mayo: Swap in 2 tablespoons of mashed avocado (45 calories) in place of 2 tablespoons of mayonnaise (180 calories) on a sandwich. The avocado has one-fourth the calories and has healthy fats, much less sodium, and more nutrition. Make this change once a week and you'll save over 7,000 calories in a year. Again, that one swap can save enough calories to lose about 2 pounds!

Swap vegetables: Swap a green salad of non-starchy vegetables in place of mashed potatoes, a starchy vegetable.

- 1 cup green salad = 50 calories, 5 grams carbohydrate
- 1 cup mashed potatoes = 240 calories, 30 grams carbohydrate

Takeaway: You could eat nearly 5 cups of salad for the calories you'd get in 1 cup of mashed potatoes! Vegetables that are not starchy are a good thing to fill up on, and they won't raise blood glucose much. See Chapter 3 for more ideas on vegetable swaps.

Swap meats: Swap a grilled, skinless chicken breast in place of a grilled pork chop.

- 4-ounce grilled pork chop = 235 calories, 10 grams fat
- 4-ounce grilled, skinless chicken breast = 187 calories, 4 grams fat

Takeaway: You could eat an extra ounce of chicken for the same calories in a pork chop and still get a lot less fat. Lean meat over fattier meat is the way to go, and it won't raise blood glucose much, if any!

Tip #2: Enjoy Your Food More, But Eat Less

Have you ever found that when eating while doing something else your attention is elsewhere and you eat more than planned? Or when you eat fast, you may eat too much and then feel overly full? I encourage you to begin to pay closer attention to hunger cues. Is your stomach growling and feeling empty? And pay attention to fullness cues while you are eating and after. Eating slower and being more mindful can help you enjoy your food more and eat less overall.

Two Strategies to Enjoy Your Food More

Take an eating "timeout." This is a strategy that has helped many of my clients. Basically, after eating for a couple of minutes, take a rest for a minute or two. Taking a rest will allow you to check in with how full you're feeling. Many people who eat quickly miss that signal and end up eating more than planned or desired.

If possible, dim the lights and listen to relaxing music. Creating a calming mood sets the tone for a slower-paced, more relaxing and enjoyable meal.

Tip #3: Downsize Portions

Putting this tip into practice can get you on your way. More managed portions means fewer calories. However, portion control doesn't mean you are destined to eat tiny amounts of everything. Just beginning to eat off smaller plates, out of smaller bowls, and drinking out of smaller cups automatically downsizes portions for you. You can learn many more tips to manage portions in Chapter 7.

Quick Portion Tip

Start your meal with a large glass of water or other zero-calorie beverage. Drinking zero-calorie fluids will help to begin to fill you up so you're more likely to be satisfied with smaller portions of food.

Which Approach Is Best for Diabetes and Weight Loss?

There are many approaches to losing weight. In fact, if you do a Google search of "how to lose weight," over 785 million entries appear! *But which weight loss approach is best for people with type 2 diabetes?* The best approach to use for weight loss is the one that enables you to keep the weight off for a lifetime. Beyond the jump-start tips just reviewed, a variety of eating patterns can help in the management of diabetes. These new approaches are much different than the message of "No concentrated sweets!" from years past. Healthful eating patterns include combinations of different nutrient-dense foods and food groups. Eating patterns include *all* foods and beverages consumed. There are eight different eating patterns acknowledged to be beneficial in managing type 2 diabetes, per the 2019 *Nutrition Therapy for Adults with Diabetes or Prediabetes: A Consensus Report:*

- Vegetarian or vegan
- Low-fat
- Very-low-fat (such as Ornish or Pritikin)
- Low-carbohydrate
- Very-low-carbohydrate
- DASH (Dietary Approach to Stop Hypertension)
- Mediterranean-style
- Paleo

The first six in particular are beneficial for weight loss. One is not clearly superior to another. Chapter 3 will discuss all of these eating patterns. Your personal preferences and goals are important considerations when choosing an eating pattern to follow. Work with your registered dietitian nutritionist to determine which eating pattern is the best for you.

Other Weight Loss Options

In addition to healthy eating, physical activity, and behavior change, other options for weight loss include the following:

Weight Loss Medications

There are weight loss medications to aid in both short-term and long-term weight management. For some people, these medications can be effective add-ons to diet, enhanced physical activity, and behavioral counseling. Weight loss medications for people with type 2 diabetes may be considered if BMI is $\geq$27 kg/m^2. Some of these medications have unpleasant side effects, and, of course, they only work when you take them. Weighing the potential benefits against possible side effects and risks is key.

Medical Devices for Weight Loss

There are several minimally invasive medical devices recently approved by the U.S. Food and Drug Administration (FDA) for short-term weight loss. These devices are very expensive and have limited coverage by insurance. They are not the standard of care in obesity management in people with type 2 diabetes.

Weight Loss Surgery (Also Called Metabolic Surgery)

Weight loss surgery *may* be an option for adults with type 2 diabetes who have BMI levels of 30.0–34.9 kg/m² (27.5–32.4 kg/m² in Asian Americans) and who have not been able to achieve weight loss and improved blood glucose levels with reasonable nonsurgical methods. Metabolic surgery *should* be recommended as an option to treat type 2 diabetes in appropriate surgical candidates with BMI levels ≥40 kg/m² (≥37.5 kg/m² in Asian Americans) and in adults with BMI levels of 35.0–39.9 kg/m² (32.5–37.4 kg/m² in Asian Americans) who do not achieve weight loss and improved associated medical conditions, including elevated blood glucose, with reasonable nonsurgical methods.

Physical Activity

Regular physical activity is a good thing! As you learned in Chapter 1, exercise has many benefits. Regular physical activity lowers blood glucose, can help with both weight loss and prevention of weight regain, helps keep the heart healthy, and is a great stress reliever. The intent here is to provide you with general guidelines. Talk with your healthcare team about whether these are safe and best for you, particularly if you have not been exercising lately.

Move More, Sit Less

The goal is to move more and sit less. You learned in the last chapter that regular physical activity is beneficial for *preventing* type 2 diabetes, but it is also hugely beneficial in *managing* type 2 diabetes. Try to move at least every 30 minutes for blood glucose benefits.

How Much Physical Activity Is Best?

The goal should be to get at least 150 minutes each week of activity that raises your heart rate. This type of activity is known as "aerobic" exercise. An example of moderate-intensity activity would be taking a brisk walk where you walk a mile in 17 minutes. If you haven't been exercising regularly, you may need to start at a slower pace or shorter distance and work your way up as your body gets stronger. Spread physical activity out over at least 3 days. And don't go more than 2 consecutive days without activity

---

Aim for 2–3 Fewer Sedentary Hours Each Day: 3 Tips to Reduce Sedentary Time

1. Every half hour, stand for 1–3 minutes.
2. When watching TV, stand up or walk around during commercials. (If you record or watch On-Demand television like me, then move around after each half-hour show.)
3. Use an app or set a reminder to move.

(to get the most benefit). Exercise has roughly a 24-hour glucose-lowering effect, so aim for at least every other day. Every 10-minute block of exercise counts!

Do You Know About the Talk Test?

To help you know if you are walking or exercising at a "just right" pace, you should be able to talk without gasping for breath, but you shouldn't be able to sing. If you can sing, it's a sign you need to pick up the pace (as your health allows).

Other Types of Helpful Exercise

Resistance Exercise

Resistance exercise is activity that causes muscles to contract against an external resistance. Examples of these activities include using resistance bands or weights or doing sit-ups, chin-ups, and pushups. You can gain additional blood glucose–lowering benefits by fitting in two to three sessions of resistance exercise each week, with each session consisting of at least one set of five or more different resistance exercises involving the large muscle groups. Again, you'll want to spread these sessions out throughout the week. Resistance exercise helps increase strength, muscle mass and tone, and endurance.

Flexibility Exercise

Flexibility training and balance training are recommended two to three times each week as well, particularly for older adults with diabetes. Yoga and tai chi are two examples that may be included to increase flexibility, muscular

strength, and balance. These types of exercise can have significant glucose-lowering impacts.

Get the Most Bang for Your Buck

I often get asked, "When is the best time to exercise?" My reply is, "Whenever you can fit it in." Ideally, you can get the most bang for your buck by exercising when your blood glucose is peaking, which is generally 1–2 hours after eating. (Because exercise generally lowers blood glucose, if you take insulin or another diabetes medication and hypoglycemia is a side effect, know the signs and carry treatment with you. Learn more about the symptoms and treatment in Chapter 4 on pages 72 and 73.)

7 Tips to Fit More Fitness Into Your Day

1. Stand up and walk around when talking on the phone.
2. March in place while watching TV.
3. Mow the lawn using a push mower.
4. Take the stairs instead of the elevator or escalator.
5. Stand at your desk rather than sit.
6. Weed, rake, and prune; gardening is an everyday way to be more active.
7. Get fit at work by doing exercises at your desk (such as doing desk pushups, walking/jogging/running in place, or doing chair squats and calf raises).

Talk with your healthcare team about what type, amount, and intensity of activity is best for you.

In addition to physical activity, healthy eating and behavior change can help you lose weight. See Table 2.3 for examples of lifestyle

TABLE 2.3   LIFESTYLE CHANGES THAT WORK FOR WEIGHT LOSS

Healthy Eating	Physical Activity	Behavior Change
Monitor your weight and blood glucose each day. It's much easier to make small, daily modifications to your food and activity level than to try to offset a larger weight gain or A1C above target.	**Aim to walk at least 10,000 steps each day.** Use an activity tracker or step counter (pedometer) to count your steps.	**Set specific and attainable goals,** such as replacing an after-dinner TV show with a walk. It can build your confidence to change your behavior for the better.
Eat less fat, and that will help you to eat fewer calories. If you swap in skim milk in place of whole milk, you'll save 56 calories for each cup. Do that three times a day, and the calorie savings translates into almost 18 pounds of weight loss over a year.	**Look for ways to increase your heart rate during your daily routine.** Take the stairs more often. Get up and walk every half hour.	**Change your eating style to make it easier to eat less without feeling deprived.** Incorporate one or more of the tips in this chapter.
Eat the rainbow. Fill half of your plate with non-starchy vegetables. Include a variety of colorful vegetables and fruits, which are packed with fiber and nutrients.	**If you don't have time to exercise 30 minutes at one time, break it up into three 10-minute sessions.** You'll still reap benefits in calorie burning and blood glucose lowering.	**Keep exercise clothes and shoes in the car or at work,** so you're prepared when an opportunity to be active arises.

Are High Lipids a Challenge for You?

The following lifestyle interventions can help lower lipids. You'll learn more about each of these as you make your way through the book. Chapter 5 contains more information on fats, fiber, and plant stanols/sterols.

- Lose weight, if overweight.
- Be more physically active.
- Adopt the DASH (Dietary Approach to Stop Hypertension) eating pattern. For prediabetes, the Mediterranean, vegetarian or vegan, and low-carbohydrate/very-low-carbohydrate eating plans may be beneficial as well.
- Eat less solid fats (saturated and trans fats).
- Eat more omega-3 fats.
- Eat more fiber.
- Eat more plant stanols and sterols.

Is High Blood Pressure a Problem for You?

The following lifestyle interventions can help lower blood pressure. Again, you'll learn about each of these as you make your way through the book.

- Lose weight, if overweight.
- Be more physically active.
- Adopt the DASH eating pattern, including reducing sodium and increasing potassium (you'll learn about DASH in Chapter 3).
- Moderate alcohol intake.

---

changes you can make to help promote weight loss.

Stress Management

How do you feel about living with diabetes? Living with diabetes can be stressful. And stress can have a big impact on your diabetes management. Stress causes your body to make hormones that raise blood glucose. When you are stressed, it is common to spend a lot of time thinking about the past and worrying about the future. It may also be harder to eat healthy, be physically active, take your medication, or check your blood glucose frequently enough. Managing stress is an important part of staying healthy with diabetes. Managing stress means either reducing stressors in your life or reducing your response to stress.

7 Tactics That Can Help Manage Stress

1. **Practice mindfulness and being present in the moment.** Mindfulness can help you not get caught up in dwelling on the past or worrying about the future.
2. **Practice an attitude of gratitude.** Each day identify at least three specific things for which you are grateful. Some may be big; some may be small. Write them down and refer back to them when you are feeling stressed or down.
3. **Identify one or more things that are going well with your diabetes management.** *How did you accomplish this success? How could you accomplish this more often?*
4. **Engage in regular physical activity.** Regular exercise helps lower the production of stress hormones and may help you sleep better.
5. **Get enough sleep.** When you are sleep-deprived, the stress response can be magnified. Turn off electronic devices, create a quiet atmosphere, take a hot shower, and avoid caffeine and alcohol in the evening to help bring sleep quicker.
6. **Practice yoga.** Many leading experts recommend yoga for diabetes management. To get started, check out the variety of yoga-for-diabetes videos and poses online.
7. **Try tai chi.** You can find a variety of guided tai-chi-for-diabetes videos online.

Tobacco Cessation

While on the topic of stress management, I want to encourage you, if you use tobacco or nicotine in any form, to take steps to stop; using tobacco products with diabetes is a harmful combination. These products worsen blood glucose levels and increase the risk of heart disease and other health complications, which may result in premature death. Many people don't realize that tobacco and smoking may actually increase the risk for developing type 2 diabetes as well.

Get Your Zzz's

Sleep loss actually can make it harder to manage blood glucose. And when you are sleep-deprived, you may let your guard down and find yourself craving high-fat, high-carbohydrate food. Aim to get at least 7–8 hours of sleep each night.

Let your healthcare team know if diabetes is magnifying your stress level and keeping you from doing what you need to do to take care of yourself.

Partner with Your Diabetes Healthcare Team

This book is designed to provide a core basic foundation and guide you in deciding what you can and are willing to do to manage diabetes. While we've covered some basics around how lifestyle changes can positively affect managing diabetes, I encourage you to really partner with your diabetes healthcare team to focus together on how to optimize a lifestyle for you. The best way to find the individualized and personalized advice you need to ensure healthy eating success is by working with a registered dietitian nutritionist (RDN) and/or certified diabetes care and education specialist (CDCES).

Registered Dietitian Nutritionist (RDN)

I encourage you to meet with an RDN for personalized guidance to suit you. This provider may also simply go by registered dietitian (RD). The credentials you'll see after the name are RDN or RD. Strong evidence supports the effectiveness of this personalized guidance (also called "medical nutrition therapy" or MNT) in improving A1C (the measure of blood glucose over time). If diabetes is new to you, several visits initially can help get you focused and feeling confident. This personalized nutrition guidance from an RDN has been demonstrated to result in significantly lowering blood glucose. Along with individualized guidance on healthy eating with diabetes, an RDN may provide advice on how to incorporate physical activity into your life as well. For a referral to an RDN, ask your physician or locate an RDN near you through the Academy of Nutrition and Dietetics website www.eatright.org.

Diabetes Care and Education Specialist

I also encourage you to partner with a diabetes care and education specialist (formerly known as a diabetes educator) to help you garner the knowledge, skills, and ability and incorporate your needs, goals, and life experiences to take the best possible care of yourself now and in the future. A credentialed diabetes care and education specialist will have one or both of

the following credentials after his or her name: CDCES or BC-ADM. Diabetes care and education specialists can help you understand basics about how to manage diabetes and can explain the effects certain diabetes medications may have on you. They can also teach you how to monitor your blood glucose, use other diabetes-related technology and devices, solve problems, and adjust emotionally to diabetes. You can ask your physician for referral to a CDCES or BC-ADM, or locate one through the Association of Diabetes Care and Education Specialists (formerly the AADE) website (www.diabeteseducator.org) or the Certification Board for Diabetes Care and Education website (www.ncbde.org). Many RDNs are also CDCESs or BC-ADMs.

How Often Should You See These Important Partners in Health?

If you're newly diagnosed with type 2 diabetes, three or four visits with an RDN can get your diabetes eating plan off to a great start. After that, a visit at least every year and during times of changing health status will help you stay on track and keep you up-to-date on the latest developments in the area of healthy eating for diabetes.

4 Critical Times to Check in with Your Diabetes Care and Education Specialist:

1. At diagnosis
2. Annually (think about it as your nutrition and diabetes education "checkup")
3. Whenever you experience complicating factors that influence your

self-management (such as other health conditions, physical limitations, emotional factors, change in your living situation, etc.)

4. When there are transitions in your care (such as a change in insurance coverage or healthcare provider, or you are now living alone)

Spending time with an RDN and/or diabetes care and education specialist is a great investment in your future. This provider can give helpful guidance and support to maintain improvements in blood glucose. These visits are generally covered benefits on most health insurance plans.

Preparing for Your Visit: What to Take with You

- ✔ Consult/referral form from your doctor's office (if not sent directly to the provider)
- ✔ Copy of the results from your most recent checkup
- ✔ Recent medical and lab test results
- ✔ Blood glucose meter or continuous glucose monitor (CGM), if you have one
- ✔ Your blood glucose log, if you have been checking your blood glucose at home, or CGM tracings
- ✔ List of all medicines and supplements you take, including the dosages
- ✔ Any nutrition information or eating plan you have received in the past or are currently following

- ✔ Any diabetes/nutrition information that you have been reading or researching
- ✔ A food journal (written or electronic) that lists everything you eat and drink in the 3–7 days before the appointment. Remember to include serving sizes and how the food was prepared. Record carbohydrate content, if possible.
- ✔ Nutrition Facts labels on products you have questions about
- ✔ A list of questions you want answered
- ✔ A report on your progress (if it's a return visit)
- ✔ A list of goals you hope to accomplish
- ✔ A friend or family member to help provide information and absorb the new information
- ✔ Your insurance card and photo identification

Putting It All Together

We touched on the AADE7 Self-Care Behaviors for managing diabetes in the Introduction. We'll revisit those now. Learning about successful diabetes management is a lifelong process. Working with your diabetes care and education specialist and diabetes healthcare team, you can use these seven Self-Care Behaviors as a checklist to be sure you've learned about every important area of diabetes self-management. Behaviors listed in Table 2.4 are based on those available on the Association of Diabetes Care and Education Specialists (formerly the AADE) website (www.diabeteseducator.org).

TABLE 2.4   AADE7 SELF-CARE BEHAVIORS FOR MANAGING DIABETES

Self-Care Behavior	Do you know . . .
Healthy Eating	• the effect of carbohydrate on blood glucose? • what, when, and how much to eat?
Being Active	• how often, how long, and at what intensity you should exercise? • how to balance physical activity with your food and medication?
Monitoring	• how often you need to check your blood glucose? • your target goals for blood glucose, blood pressure, and blood lipids?
Taking Medication	• the names, doses, and actions of your medications? • the side effects of your medications?
Problem Solving	• the symptoms of hyperglycemia (high blood glucose) and hypoglycemia (low blood glucose)? • how to adjust your food, medication, and physical activity based on your blood glucose levels?
Reducing Risks	• which tests and exams will enable you to better monitor your health? • how to prevent the complications of diabetes?
Healthy Coping	• the benefits of diabetes self-care? • how to find support for dealing with diabetes?

Other Resources

American Diabetes Association's Website

You can also learn more about managing all aspects of your diabetes or prediabetes by going to the American Diabetes Association's website (www.diabetes.org). The website is brimming with food tips, meal-planning tools, shopping lists, and recipes, as well as a guide to healthy eating and physical activity that can lead to improved blood glucose management. You can also visit the Association's dedicated food and cooking website, Diabetes Food Hub (www.diabetesfoodhub. org), to find recipes and plan your meals.

USDA "Choose My Plate" Website

The U.S. Department of Agriculture (USDA) also has a wealth of no-cost information about healthy eating for the general public as well as meal plans for weight loss on the Choose My Plate website (www.choosemyplate.gov). While not diabetes-specific, this online resource includes guidance on what to eat and drink along with personalized MyPlate Plans and tips for making better food choices while at home or eating out.

Books

If you are interested in reading a good book about diabetes or prediabetes, all of the following titles are available at www.shopdiabetes.org.

- *Prediabetes: A Complete Guide* by Jill Weisenberger, MS, RDN, CDE, CHWC, FAND
- *The Diabetes 2-Month Turnaround* by Laura Hieronymus, DNP, MLDE, BC-ADM, CDE, and Stacy Griffin, PharmD, LDE, CPT
- *Your Type 2 Diabetes Action Plan* by the American Diabetes Association

Healthy Eating for a Lifetime: It Starts with a Single Step

Without a doubt, there is definitely more than one way to eat healthy. Healthy eating is about what works for you, your life, and your health. And it's your eating style over time that matters most. The intent of this book is to help you find your healthy eating style to help manage blood glucose. In Chapter 3, you will learn how to fill and portion your plate based on an eating pattern that helps you achieve your health goals and that works for you. We'll focus on many small switches and changes to help you head in the right direction and make healthier choices you can enjoy. It's been said that whoever wants to reach a distant goal must take small steps. Small steps lead to big achievements.

Next Steps

1. Identify one swap you can make to trim calories.
2. Identify one way you can fit more movement or steps into your day.
3. Identify one tactic you can try to help manage stress.

Food for Thought

- Changing lifestyle is a journey, not a sprint.
- Lifestyle change is a process that begins with small steps, small swaps, and small changes in what you eat, how you manage weight, how you move, and how you manage stress.
- Partner with your healthcare team, registered dietitian nutritionist, and diabetes care and education specialist to get guidance and support on how to optimize a lifestyle for you.

BUILDING BLOCKS, EATING PATTERNS, AND THE DIABETES PLATE METHOD

Everything you eat and drink over time matters. The right mix can help you be healthier now and in the future. It's important to find what works for you and your family within your food preferences, health goals, and budget. Small changes can lead to healthier choices you can enjoy.

In Chapter 2, you learned about the general *Dietary Guidelines for Americans* (DGA), which give perspective and a place to start as you embrace eating healthy. And you learned about MyPlate, which illustrates what a healthy meal looks like based on the DGA. In this chapter, we will build on that and learn about the eight different eating patterns that can benefit blood glucose and lower cardiovascular risk factors. We will also learn how to portion your plate for diabetes.

Building Blocks

Foods are composed of three basic nutrients that nourish the body:

- Carbohydrates
- Fats
- Proteins

You can think of these as building blocks that supply calories along with other nutrients. Your body needs all three to be healthy.

3 Things You Need to Know:

1. Carbohydrate gets the most attention when it comes to diabetes because carbohydrate is the component of your meals and snacks

33

that is *most directly responsible for the rise in blood glucose after eating.* Carbohydrate is found in grains, beans, and other starchy foods; fruit; milk/dairy and milk substitutes; nonstarchy vegetables (however, in much lesser amounts); sweetened beverages; and sweet treats. You'll learn much more about carbohydrate in Chapter 4.

2. Protein and fat do not affect postprandial (after-eating) blood glucose to anywhere near the extent that carbohydrate does, particularly in people with type 2 diabetes or prediabetes. Protein-rich foods include meat, poultry, fish, seafood, and eggs. You'll learn much more about protein foods in Chapter 5.

3. Fat is most concentrated in calories, providing more than twice the calories of protein or carbohydrate. You can cut out a lot of calories simply by eating less fat and fatty foods.

Let's look at an example: Swap 1 tablespoon of spicy mustard in place of 1 tablespoon of mayonnaise on a sandwich. Save about 90 calories and 15 grams of fat. Make that swap twice a week, and save 9,360 calories and 1,560 grams of fat in 1 year. That's a savings equal to 13 sticks of butter!

With that said, we don't eat these individual building blocks alone; we eat foods that are a combination of them. And there is not a one-size-fits-all ideal combination or distribution of carbohydrate, protein, and fat. However, there are actually a variety of eating *patterns* that are beneficial in managing diabetes.

Eating Patterns

What is an eating pattern? An eating pattern is basically a combination of different foods, food groups, and beverages consumed. Evidence shows that a variety of eating patterns can help manage diabetes.

As you learned in Chapter 2, there are eight different eating patterns acknowledged to be beneficial in managing type 2 diabetes:

- Vegetarian or vegan
- Low-fat
- Very-low-fat (such as Ornish or Pritikin)
- Low-carbohydrate
- Very-low-carbohydrate
- DASH (Dietary Approach to Stop Hypertension)
- Mediterranean-style
- Paleo

No one pattern has emerged as being superior to the others. The first six in particular are beneficial for weight loss. The low-carbohydrate and very-low-carbohydrate patterns have demonstrated the most evidence for lowering blood glucose, so if you have blood glucose above target or want to reduce diabetes medications, adopting a low- or very-low-carbohydrate eating pattern will help.

Mediterranean is the main eating pattern that has reported reduced risk of major cardiovascular events. Vegetarian or vegan, low-fat, low-carbohydrate/very-low-carbohydrate, and DASH eating patterns have demonstrated cardiovascular-protective benefits. Your registered dietitian nutritionist can provide much more in-depth information on the specific cardio-protective benefits of each.

Key factors that are common among these eating patterns:

- Emphasize nonstarchy vegetables
- Minimize added sugar and refined grains
- Emphasize choosing whole foods over highly processed foods to the extent possible

Your personal preferences and goals are important considerations when choosing an eating pattern to embrace. After you learn more about these eating patterns in this chapter, consider your personal preferences and goals and which eating pattern you may want to try. Then, work with your registered dietitian nutritionist to determine which eating pattern is best for you, and if you could benefit from an individualized eating plan. This eating plan would guide when, what, and how much to eat each day of the foods in your selected eating pattern, factoring in your calorie and carbohydrate goals.

You read about the *Dietary Guidelines for Americans* (DGA) in Chapter 2. Below is a summary for comparison as you review the eating patterns that follow.

USDA Dietary Guidelines for Americans:

- Emphasizes a variety of vegetables from all of the subgroups
- Emphasizes fruit, especially whole fruit
- Includes grains with at least half being whole grains
- Incorporates lower-fat dairy
- Includes a variety of protein foods
- Includes oils instead of solid fats
- Limits saturated fats, trans fats, added sugars, and sodium

Vegetarian or Vegan (Plant-Based) Eating Pattern

Focused around plant foods, the plant-based eating pattern often results in weight loss and lower blood glucose and LDL cholesterol. Plant-based eating means eating more fruits, vegetables, whole grains, nuts, and soy products (Table 3.1). This eating pattern is rich in "good" fiber, vitamins, minerals, phytochemicals (healthy plant compounds), and healthy fats. These foods are low in the "bad" saturated fat and cholesterol.

Plant Power Formula

If your goal is to eat more plant-based foods, try using the plant power "formula," a method I use when pulling together a plant-based meal.

TABLE 3.1   FACTS AND FOODS FOR A VEGETARIAN OR VEGAN EATING PATTERN

Vegetarian or Vegan Eating Pattern	Description	Sample Meal Ideas
Revolves around plant-based foods	• Focused around plant-based foods (such as vegetables, beans, nuts and seeds, fruit, whole grains, soy and other plant-based products) • **Vegetarian approach** (also known as lacto-ovo vegetarian) excludes animal flesh foods but includes eggs (ovo) and/or dairy (lacto) products • **Vegan approach** excludes any animal products or flesh foods • Rich in fiber and phyto-chemicals (healthy plant compounds)	**Vegetarian** **Breakfast:** Egg scrambled with onion, red pepper, and spinach; slice of toasted whole-grain bread spread with mashed avocado or hummus; tomato or vegetable juice **Lunch:** Kale salad with quinoa, pomegranate seeds, mandarin orange sections, mukimame (shelled edamame/soybeans), walnuts, vinaigrette **Dinner:** Black bean burger with lettuce, tomato, onion, on 100% whole-wheat bun; sautéed zucchini, mushrooms, tomatoes, and artichokes; milk **Snacks:** Smoothie made with Greek yogurt, unsweetened frozen fruit, and almond or soy milk **Vegan** **Breakfast:** Vegan 100% whole-grain seeded bread, toasted, topped with almond butter, sliced strawberries, blueberries, and unsalted sunflower seeds; almond or soy milk **Lunch:** Vegan tomato basil soup topped with pan-cooked tempeh; small plum **Dinner:** Tofu stir-fried with broccoli, snow peas, water chestnuts, mushrooms, and baby corn over farro **Snacks:** Pumpkin seeds, soy nuts, dried cherries

Using this formula, you can pull together a multitude of delicious, wholesome options. Here's how it works:

1. Choose a whole grain.
2. Add a plant protein (such as beans, lentils, tofu, or nuts).
3. Add a fruit or vegetable.

Applying the plant power formula at breakfast:

1. Choose a whole grain: steel-cut oats.
2. Add a plant protein: toasted almonds.
3. Add a fruit or vegetable: blueberries and raspberries.

Applying the plant power formula at lunch:

1. Choose a whole grain: quinoa.
2. Add a plant protein: chickpeas or lentils.
3. Add a fruit or vegetable: kale, tomatoes, broccoli; then drizzle with olive oil vinaigrette.

Applying the plant power formula at dinner:

1. Choose a whole grain: brown rice.
2. Add a plant protein: veggie chili with beans over the rice.
3. Add a fruit or vegetable: fresh strawberries.

Vitamin B12: A Special Consideration

Vitamin B12 in not naturally found in plant foods. Most vegetarians are not deficient in vitamin B12 if they consume milk, cheese, eggs, and fortified foods. However, vegans should consider discussing with their doctor or registered dietitian nutritionist the options for increasing vitamin B12 consumption (usually with supplementation, fortified foods, and/or sometimes using nutritional yeast).

Embrace a More Plant-Based Eating Pattern 1 Meal, 1 Day, 1 Week at a Time

- Make beans, lentils, or soy products the focus of your meals. While adding variety, this will also save money because these protein sources cost less than meat, poultry, and fish.
- Begin the week with "meatless Mondays," such as with a black bean soup for lunch or dinner.
- Add in a vegetarian breakfast with whole-grain cereal, almond milk, and half of a banana.
- Give a favorite recipe a plant-based makeover. (See more recipe renewal ideas in Chapter 11.)

Three swaps to live a little more plant-based:

1. Try plant-based "dairy" products such as unsweetened almond milk or soy milk. Read the Nutrition Facts label and look for no sugar added. These products are an easy swap in most recipes.
2. Swap cooked lentils in place of ground beef in tacos, sloppy joes, or Shepherd's pie.
3. Swap black beans in place of pork, chicken, or ground beef in burritos or enchiladas.

Items to stock up on to live a little more plant-based:

- **Fresh vegetables:** Carrots, celery, beets, bell peppers, and onions have a longer shelf-life than some other vegetables and can be used in a variety of recipes. Fresh greens are good for a quick salad, sautéing, steaming, or tossing in scrambles, soups, or stews.

- **Fresh fruits:** Apples, clementines, grapes, oranges, and pears last a long time in the fridge and make quick snacks.
- **Nuts and seeds:** Almonds, cashews, peanuts, pistachios, and walnuts are a few ideas. If you buy in bulk, store extras in the freezer in zip-top freezer bags to keep them from spoiling, and pull them out as you need them.
- **Plant-based milk:** Almond, rice, or soy are options to keep on hand.
- **Condiments:** Salsa and/or hot sauce can spice up the flavor.
- **Hummus:** Dunk vegetables in hummus or spread on a sandwich.
- **Nut butters or tahini:** Spread on toast and sandwiches or use in dressings.
- **Freezer staples:** These staples can include frozen plain vegetables, frozen unsweetened fruit, cooked whole grains, cooked beans, and whole-wheat or corn tortillas. I often cook extra beans and grains and freeze portions in 1-cup containers to pull out and incorporate into meals.

Low-Fat Eating Pattern

Low-fat eating patterns are typically described as containing no more than 30% of total calories from fat. In my experience, when people embrace a low-fat eating pattern, they often begin buying foods labeled "fat-free" or "low-fat," when in fact wholesome vegetables, fruits, whole grains, lean protein, and low-fat dairy are naturally lower in fat (see Table 3.2). The low-fat eating pattern emphasizes these wholesome foods rather than low-fat processed foods.

Let's Do the Math for an Average 1,800 Calories

- No more than 30% of calories from fat means no more than 60 grams of total fat each day.

  1,800 calories × 0.30 = 540 calories divided by 9 calories per gram of fat = 60 grams of total fat

- No more than 10% of calories from saturated fat means no more than 20 grams of saturated fat each day.

  1,800 calories × 0.10 = 180 calories divided by 9 calories per gram of fat = 20 grams of saturated fat

---

Note: 1,800 calories is used simply as an illustration. Talk with your registered dietitian nutritionist about the amount that is best for you. Until then, to get a general idea, check out the calorie counter at choosemyplate.gov.

Very-Low-Fat Eating Pattern

Two of the most well-known very-low-fat eating patterns are the Pritikin diet and Ornish diet. The Ornish diet emphasizes real foods as

TABLE 3.2   FACTS AND FOODS FOR A LOW-FAT EATING PATTERN

Low-Fat Eating Pattern	Description	Sample Meal Ideas
≤30% of total calories coming from fat ≤10% of total calories coming from saturated fat	• Emphasizes vegetables (nonstarchy and starchy), fruits, whole grains, and other starches (such as breads/crackers, pasta) • Includes lean proteins (including beans) • Includes low-fat dairy products	**Breakfast:** Egg white scramble with tomato and basil in a whole-wheat tortilla; small banana; nonfat milk **Lunch:** Vegetable soup; turkey on whole-grain seeded bread with mustard, lettuce, tomato, cucumber; cherries **Dinner:** Shrimp and vegetable stir-fry over riced cauliflower; fresh pineapple **Snacks:** Low-fat popcorn; kiwi

they're found in nature rather than processed foods. This plan is a very-low-fat, plant-based, whole-food approach and provides around 60 grams of fiber daily (that's a lot!). The very-low-fat Pritikin diet intervention is high in fiber and focuses on plant-based foods. The Pritikin program is provided during an inpatient treatment center stay and includes personalized exercise programs, stress management, one-on-one counseling, and education programs. Table 3.3 discusses low-fat food options and sample meal ideas.

Suggestions through the day to swap out fat and swap in fiber to fill you up:

- At breakfast, swap in oats in place of granola cereal.
- At lunch, swap in hummus on a whole-grain sandwich rather than mayonnaise.
- At dinner, swap in beans for meat.
- At snacks, swap in roasted chickpeas or edamame in place of nuts.

Low-Carbohydrate Eating Pattern

The low-carbohydrate and very-low-carbohydrate eating patterns described on the next page have demonstrated blood glucose–lowering power, reducing both A1C and the need for glucose-lowering medication. These are among the most studied eating patterns for type 2 diabetes. As you'll see, low-carbohydrate eating patterns focus on foods higher in protein, healthy fats, and vegetables that are low in carbohydrate (Table 3.4). Fruit and higher-carbohydrate vegetables can be worked in; however, added sugar–containing foods and grain products are often very limited or avoided altogether.

TABLE 3.3 FACTS AND FOODS FOR A VERY-LOW-FAT EATING PATTERN

Very-Low-Fat Eating Pattern	Description	Sample Meal Ideas
10% of total calories coming from fat For an average 1,800 calories, that means less than 20 grams of fat each day.	• Emphasizes fiber-rich vegetables (nonstarchy and starchy), beans, fruits, whole grains, nonfat dairy • Is rich in carbohydrate foods, with focus on unprocessed foods • Is high in fiber (30–60 grams daily) • Emphasizes fish and egg whites	**Breakfast:** Steel-cut oats with cinnamon and raisins, nonfat milk **Lunch:** Navy bean soup; arugula or spinach with vinaigrette; fresh raspberries **Dinner:** Grilled chicken over black beans and brown rice topped with diced avocado and fresh salsa **Snacks:** Pear; edamame

TABLE 3.4 FACTS AND FOODS FOR A LOW-CARBOHYDRATE EATING PATTERN

Low-Carbohydrate Eating Pattern	Description	Sample Meal Ideas
There is not a consistent definition of "low carbohydrate," but the amount of carbohydrate eaten is moderately low (26–45% of total daily calories).	• Emphasizes nonstarchy vegetables • Emphasizes protein from meat, poultry, fish, shellfish, eggs, cheese, nuts, and seeds • Uses fats from animal foods, oils, butter, avocado • Some people choose to include fruit • Avoids starchy and sugary foods (such as pasta, rice, potatoes, bread, and sweets)	**Breakfast:** Steel-cut oats with almond or peanut butter stirred in; boiled or scrambled egg (or egg substitute) **Lunch:** Turkey caprese wrap: small whole-wheat tortilla filled with smoked turkey, sliced tomato, slice of fresh mozzarella, fresh basil leaves (or pesto); grapes **Dinner:** Grilled chicken breast, roasted Brussels sprouts, small baked sweet potato topped with trans-fat-free margarine, cinnamon, and toasted pecans **Snacks**: Apple slices spread with low-fat cottage cheese and sprinkled with cinnamon; unsalted or lightly salted almonds

There doesn't seem to be a consistent definition of "low carbohydrate," but the amount of carbohydrate eaten may range from low, with about one-quarter to just under half the calories coming from carbohydrate foods (26–45% of total calories), to very low carbohydrate, with a goal of around 20–50 grams of non-fiber carbohydrate each day (which is less than 26% of total calories). You'll learn much more about carbohydrate and tips on how to reduce carbohydrate in Chapter 4. And you'll learn more about fiber in Chapter 5.

A low- or very-low-carbohydrate eating plan is *not* recommended for people with kidney disease, women who are pregnant or breastfeeding, people struggling with eating disorders, or people taking a type of diabetes medicine called an SGLT2 (sodium–glucose cotransporter 2) inhibitor because of the potential risk for serious health problems.

Refer to Chapter 4 for lots of practical tips on reducing carbohydrate.

Very-Low-Carbohydrate Eating Pattern

While carbohydrate is your body's preferred fuel, one can adapt to burning fat rather than carbohydrate as the primary fuel. A very-low-carbohydrate eating pattern typically includes only 20–50 grams of non-fiber carbohydrate each day (fiber doesn't raise blood glucose) (see Table 3.5). Reducing carbohydrate this drastically can cause you to get rid of a lot of fluid and swiftly lower blood glucose. Thus, it is important to consult with your diabetes healthcare team if you are considering this eating pattern, to help prevent dehydration and to possibly reduce diabetes medications to prevent blood glucose from dropping too low.

Sustaining a very-low-carbohydrate approach can be challenging. Assessing what is doable and individualizing it to suit your needs is key, since individuals have different "tolerances" for carbohydrate.

DASH Eating Pattern

DASH stands for Dietary Approaches to Stop Hypertension. This eating pattern has helped individuals improve blood pressure and lower diabetes risk as well as lose weight. The DASH pattern is rich in vegetables, fruits, low-fat or nonfat dairy, whole grains, poultry, fish,

---

Let's Do the Math for an Average 1,800 Calories

For an average 1,800 calories, carbohydrates would total between 117 and 203 grams a day (or **34–63 grams per meal if split evenly between meals with one 15-gram carbohydrate snack**).

1,800 calories × 0.26 = 468 calories divided by 4 calories per gram of carbohydrate = 117 grams of carbohydrate

1,800 calories × 0.45 = 810 calories divided by 4 calories per gram of carbohydrate = 203 grams of carbohydrate

TABLE 3.5   FACTS AND FOODS FOR A VERY-LOW-CARBOHYDRATE EATING PATTERN

Very-Low-Carbohydrate Eating Pattern	Description	Sample Meal Ideas
Typically contains only 20–50 grams of non-fiber carbohydrate each day	• Similar to the low-carbohydrate pattern, but further limits carbohydrate-containing foods • Meals are typically high in fat with more than half of the calories coming from fat	**Breakfast:** Veggie omelet or scramble with low-fat cheese and topped with diced avocado; fresh blackberries and raspberries with a dollop of Greek yogurt **Lunch:** Green salad with tuna or salmon (foil packs for ease), sliced almonds, vinaigrette dressing **Dinner:** Turkey meatballs and marinara over zucchini spirals sprinkled with parmesan cheese; chopped romaine with light Caesar salad dressing **Snacks:** String cheese; peanuts; cucumber slices with salsa for dipping

and nuts. This plan is low in sodium, added sugar, and solid saturated fat. As you can see in Table 3.6, the DASH eating pattern is heavily plant-based. This diet is much lower in fat and includes more dairy than the Mediterranean eating pattern.

5 Tips to Transition to a DASH-Style Eating Pattern

(Specific examples of the foods mentioned below follow later in the chapter.)

1. **Begin to work in more nonstarchy vegetables.** Add one nonstarchy vegetable in at lunch one day and at dinner the next.

2. **Add a fresh fruit at one meal or as a snack.**

3. **Add in a fat-free or low-fat dairy product until you're up to three a day.** Examples of these foods could be low-fat milk at breakfast, a Greek yogurt for lunch, and kefir or drinkable yogurt for a snack.

4. **Limit meat to a portion the size of a deck of cards twice a day.** If you eat more than that, gradually reduce

TABLE 3.6 FACTS AND FOODS FOR A DASH EATING PATTERN

DASH Eating Pattern	Description	Sample Meal Ideas
"DASH" stands for Dietary Approaches to Stop Hypertension. It is designed to help lower blood pressure by emphasizing plant foods, and reducing fat and sodium intake.	<ul><li>Emphasizes vegetables, fruits, and low-fat dairy products</li><li>Includes whole grains</li><li>Includes lean proteins such as poultry, fish, and nuts</li><li>Is reduced in saturated fat, red meat, sweets, and sugar-containing beverages</li></ul>	**Breakfast:** Whole-grain cereal with low-fat milk, blueberries, and sliced almonds **Lunch:** Salad greens topped with grilled chicken, cucumber, tomato, no-salt-added canned white beans, avocado, walnuts, and vinaigrette; clementine **Dinner:** Lemon garlic shrimp over quinoa; sautéed spinach or kale; small whole-grain roll with trans-fat-free margarine; sliced strawberries with a dollop of low-fat vanilla Greek yogurt **Snacks:** Unsalted pistachios; sliced pear sprinkled with cinnamon

portion sizes by one-third or one-half at each meal.

5. **Incorporate a meatless meal twice a week.** This meal could be something like a nut butter sandwich on whole-grain bread, a pasta primavera with whole-grain pasta, or a vegetarian chili.

4 Tips to Eat Less Sodium

1. **Keep salt out of view and off the kitchen counter and table.** If you feel the need to shake a seasoning onto foods, use a salt-free herb blend (such as Mrs. Dash).

2. **Cut back on salt a little at a time.** Your taste for salt will lessen over time (for many, in as little as a week).

3. **Be careful with condiments.** Foods like ketchup, pickles, soy sauce, and many salad dressings are high in sodium.

4. **Go for fresh.** Most of the sodium we eat is in processed foods. Fresh, close-to-nature foods are generally lower in sodium.

Mediterranean-Style Eating Pattern

The Mediterranean-style eating pattern is linked to a lower risk of type 2 diabetes, along with improved blood glucose and weight, and a reduced risk of heart attack and stroke. This eating plan is not low-fat but is rich in monounsaturated fat (heart-healthy fat) from plant sources such as olives and nuts. It can be an effective alternative to a low-fat, relatively high-carbohydrate diet. There is no one "right" way to follow the Mediterranean-style eating pattern, since there are many countries around the Mediterranean Sea, and people in the different areas eat different foods. Rather, consider the information in Table 3.7 as general guidelines.

10 Ways to Eat More Mediterranean

1. Replace butter and margarine with healthful oils such as olive or canola oil. Use these oils for cooking, dip bread in flavored olive oil, or lightly spread olive oil on whole-grain breads.

2. Choose protein foods such as skinless chicken and turkey, fish, beans, nuts,

TABLE 3.7   FACTS AND FOODS FOR A MEDITERRANEAN-STYLE EATING PATTERN

Mediterranean-Style Eating Pattern	Description	Sample Meal Ideas
Traditional Mediterranean meals feature foods grown all around the Mediterranean Sea. This eating style is easily adaptable to today's busy lifestyle.	• Emphasizes plant-based foods (such as vegetables, beans, nuts and seeds, fruit, and whole grains) • Includes fish and other seafood • Uses olive oil as the main dietary fat • Includes dairy products (mainly yogurt and cheese) in low to moderate amounts • Includes fewer than four eggs per week • Uses red meat in small amounts and limited frequency • Includes fresh herbs and spices for flavor • Includes wine in low to moderate amounts • Water is the go-to beverage • Uses concentrated sugars or honey infrequently	**Breakfast:** Greek yogurt topped with chopped figs and unsalted pistachios **Lunch:** Whole-wheat pita stuffed with hummus, salad greens, tuna dressed with olive oil and fresh lemon juice; date stuffed with almond butter **Dinner:** Grilled fish; tomato, cucumber, olive, and feta salad; lentils; watermelon; glass of red wine (if you choose to drink wine) **Snacks:** Nectarine or peach; walnuts or almonds

and other plant-based protein sources. Substitute fish and poultry for red meat. When red meats are eaten, choose lean cuts and keep portions small (about the size of a deck of cards).

3. Eat fish at least twice each week. Fresh or water-packed tuna, salmon, trout, mackerel, and herring are good choices.

4. Aim for three to five servings of vegetables each day.

5. Choose whole-grain breads and cereals, as well as whole-grain pasta and rice products.

6. Season meals with herbs and spices rather than salt.

7. Snack on nuts or seeds instead of snack foods. Keep almonds, cashews, pistachios, and walnuts on hand for quick snacks. Try tahini (sesame seed paste) as a dip or spread for bread.

8. Enjoy fruit to satisfy a sweet tooth.

9. Eat small portions of cheese or yogurt.

10. If you drink alcohol, consume a moderate amount with a meal (no more than one glass for women or two glasses for men).

6 Simple Swaps to Healthy Mediterranean-Style Fats

1. Top whole-grain toast with almond butter or peanut butter rather than butter. Natural nut butter is best (rather than the kind with added fat). If you have trouble with the nut butter

separating, screw the lid on tightly and store the jar upside down. When you turn it right-side-up to open it, the oil will be in the bottom rather than on the top.

2. Try almond milk on your morning cereal rather than dairy.

3. Mash and spread avocado on a sandwich rather than mayonnaise.

4. Add crunch to a salad with almonds, pecans, pistachios, pumpkin seeds, toasted sesame seeds, or sunflower seeds instead of bacon or croutons.

5. Lightly dip crusty bread in olive oil rather than slathering it with butter.

6. Choose olives over cheese for a snack or happy hour.

4 Mediterranean-Style Whole Grains

1. **Barley.** Barley can be used in salads, as a breakfast cereal with fruit and nuts, as a side with onions and garlic, and in soups.

2. **Bulgur.** Bulgur cooks quickly and can be enjoyed in salads. Tabbouleh salad made with tomatoes, cucumbers, garlic, fresh parsley, mint, lemon juice, and olive oil is delicious!

3. **Couscous.** Couscous has a neutral flavor, a fine texture, cooks quickly, and becomes fluffy when cooked. Enjoy it as a side dish in place of rice. Serve stews or roasted vegetables over it.

4. **Farro.** Farro is rich in fiber and protein and makes a great side dish or addition to soups and salads.

Vegetables Common to the Mediterranean Eating Pattern

Vegetables are a staple of the Mediterranean eating pattern. Cooked vegetables are often drizzled with olive oil and sometimes a squeeze of lemon. Mediterranean-style vegetables include the following: artichokes, arugula, beets, broccoli, Brussels sprouts, cabbage, carrots, celeriac, celery, chicory, cucumbers, eggplant, fennel, greens, leeks, mushrooms, nettles, okra, onions, peas, peppers, potatoes, radishes, rutabaga, scallions, shallots, sweet potatoes, tomatoes, turnip, and zucchini.

Fruits Common to the Mediterranean Eating Pattern

Whole fresh fruit is the ever-present "sweet treat." Mediterranean-style fruits include the following: apples, apricots, avocado, cherries, clementines, dates, figs, grapefruit, grapes, melons, nectarines, oranges, peaches, pears, pomegranates, strawberries, and tangerines.

4 Tips on How to Eat More Mediterranean-Style When Dining Out

Of course, dining at a Greek or Mediterranean restaurant is the easy answer. If that's not an option, here are four tips to make most restaurant meals work:

1. Choose fish or seafood as your main dish.
2. Order a side of nonstarchy vegetables, beans, or lentils.
3. Ask that olive oil be used for any fat required in the dish.
4. Choose whole-grain bread from the bread basket if you opt for bread, and then dip the bread in olive oil instead of spreading it with butter.

Paleo Eating Pattern

The paleo eating pattern is also known as the Stone Age or "caveman" diet. Research is limited around this eating pattern, although many people still choose to follow a paleo eating pattern and on a personal level may feel that they are seeing success.

The focus is on foods that would have been eaten by the hunter-gatherer cavemen. The eating pattern emphasizes lean meat, fish and shellfish, vegetables, eggs, nuts, and berries and does not include grains, dairy, salt, and sugar (Table 3.8). The fats are largely healthy fats. There is no "one way" to eat paleo. This eating pattern is based largely on eating close-to-nature "real" food.

5 Paleo-Style Swaps

1. Swap in riced cauliflower in place of rice or brown rice (which is a grain).
2. Instead of noodles, try spiralized zucchini or yellow squash or spaghetti squash (many groceries sell spiralized vegetables, or you can purchase an inexpensive spiralizer for home use).
3. Instead of peanut butter (peanuts are a legume), swap in almond butter.
4. Swap in finely chopped vegetables (such as carrots, bell peppers, onions, and mushrooms) in place of beans.

TABLE 3.8   FACTS AND FOODS FOR A PALEO EATING PATTERN

Paleo Eating Pattern	Description	Sample Meal Ideas
Emphasizes foods presumed to have been the only foods available to or consumed by humans during the Paleolithic era (hence the name "paleo").	• Emphasizes lean meat, fish, shellfish, vegetables, eggs, nuts, and berries • Avoids grains, dairy, salt, refined fats, and sugar	**Breakfast:** Stir-fried broccoli slaw topped with "fried" egg cooked in nonstick skillet; diced mango and strawberries sprinkled with chia seed **Lunch:** Salad with rotisserie chicken, dried cranberries, pecans, apple slices, and vinaigrette **Dinner:** Grilled or baked salmon, sautéed zucchini with red and yellow peppers; roasted butternut squash **Snacks:** Blueberry-banana chia smoothie made with almond milk; roasted chickpeas

5. Swap in crunchy fresh vegetables such as carrot or celery sticks in place of crackers.

How to Begin Adopting an Eating Pattern

While all of the eight eating patterns can be beneficial, which are of interest to you? Which seem to align with your preferences and priorities?

Based on what current research shows, here's when you might choose one eating pattern over another:

- **If you have prediabetes:** Choose Mediterranean, vegetarian or vegan, low-fat, or DASH.

- **If you are trying to lose weight:** Choose vegetarian or vegan, low-fat or very-low-fat, low-carbohydrate or very-low-carbohydrate, or DASH.

- **If you are trying to improve lipids:** Choose Mediterranean, vegetarian or vegan, low-carbohydrate, or very-low-carbohydrate.

- **If you are trying to lower blood pressure:** Choose very-low-fat, low-carbohydrate or very-low-carbohydrate, or DASH.

- **If you are struggling with lowering blood glucose/A1C:** Choose Mediterranean, vegetarian or vegan, or low-carbohydrate or very-low-carbohydrate.

- **If you want to reduce the risk of major cardiovascular events:** Choose Mediterranean.

Once you've decided on an eating pattern, try to spread your eating out over three meals and one or two snacks (if needed). Spreading out your eating will help to satisfy your hunger and keep blood glucose levels steady. You'll learn more about this in Chapter 4.

> **Tip:** In adopting a new-to-you eating pattern, start with one meal, 1 day each week. You don't have to overhaul everything at one time. That can feel overwhelming. Small changes add up and make a difference.

Putting Healthy Eating into Practice with the Diabetes Plate Method

What you eat has a big impact on blood glucose, weight, and overall health. Making healthy food choices can help. This process begins with how you portion your plate. Chapter 2 introduced the *Dietary Guidelines for Americans* and how these guidelines are translated into something doable through MyPlate. MyPlate tends to have a little too much carbohydrate for many people with diabetes. With a few small adjustments, MyPlate can become a healthy plate for managing diabetes. The Diabetes Plate Method is a great place to start to embrace a new eating pattern and manage

portions. Some people may be able to achieve their blood glucose, weight, and other health goals with the Diabetes Plate Method alone.

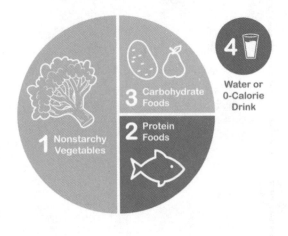

Here's How to Plan Your Portions and Create a Diabetes Plate Method Plate:

A 9-inch plate is about the right size. While many think first about the meat or protein, vegetables (the nonstarchy kind) become the focus with the Diabetes Plate Method. Nonstarchy vegetables are low in calories and don't have much effect on blood glucose. Imagine a line down the middle of the plate. Then on one side, cut it again with a horizontal line so you will have three sections on your plate.

Step #1: Fill half of your plate with nonstarchy vegetables. These vegetables include salad greens, broccoli, green beans, carrots, and tomatoes (there is a more extensive list in this chapter on page 50).

- Vary your vegetables.

Step #2: Fill one-quarter of your plate with protein. Protein foods include fish, chicken, turkey, lean beef, pork, or tofu.

- Vary your protein routine.

Step #3: Fill one-quarter of your plate with carbohydrate foods such as grains, starchy vegetables, fruit, or milk/yogurt. If your meal plan allows, you can add a glass of milk or serving of another carbohydrate food, such as fruit, outside of your plate as well.

- Focus on whole fruits instead of juice or processed fruit.
- Try to include whole grains as much as possible, such as brown rice, quinoa, barley, or bulgur.

- Make the move to low-fat and fat-free milk and yogurt.

Step #4: Choose water or another zero-calorie drink (such as unsweetened tea, sparkling water, or an occasional diet lemonade or diet soda).

Step #5: Choose healthy fats. (There is more on healthy fats to come later in this chapter and in Chapter 5.)

The Diabetes Plate Method is an easy way to plan meals. This method doesn't require any counting or too much thinking. You can create a balanced meal using the Diabetes Plate Method at home, at work, and when you go out to eat. One of the questions I've gotten

How Does a "Combination Food" Fit?

Let's use a thin-crust vegetable pizza as the example. Say you ate two slices of a medium pizza. Let's break it down and figure out how it follows the Diabetes Plate Method.

- **What kinds of foods go into it?** Flour (grain) in the crust, peppers, onions, tomatoes, tomato sauce, olives, mushrooms, and cheese
- **What parts of the plate would they go on?**
  - Peppers, onions, tomatoes, tomato sauce, olives, mushrooms: Nonstarchy vegetable half of the plate
  - Cheese: Protein quarter of the plate
  - Flour (grain) in the crust: Carbohydrate foods quarter of the plate
- **How much of the plate would they take up?** They'd all be pretty close to filling the plate if following the Diabetes Plate Method, except for the nonstarchy vegetables, which may fall a little short of filling half the plate.
- **What are a few foods you could add to fill in those sections when eating pizza?** A couple of ideas are adding a side green salad or extra veggie toppings.

frequently over the years is, "How high can you pile your plate?" A great question! The answer is no higher than a deck of cards is thick. That will help keep portions in check.

You see that sweet treats are not part of the Diabetes Plate Method. Sweets are not off limits. But fewer added sugars are best for anyone, whether they have diabetes or not. You'll learn more in Chapter 4 on carbohydrates and how to fit in occasional sweet treats.

Breaking Down the Plate: Ideas on How to Fill Each Section

Vegetables: Nonstarchy and Starchy

Vegetables are something many Americans fall short on. There are both nonstarchy vegetables and starchy vegetables. It's important to know the difference. Nonstarchy vegetables are low in calories and carbohydrates, and high in vitamins, minerals, and fiber. They only have about 25 calories for a 1/2-cup serving if cooked or a 1-cup serving if raw. Fill half your plate with nonstarchy vegetables to make sure you are getting enough servings of these nutrient-dense foods.

Starchy vegetables are also a good source of vitamins, minerals, and fiber, but they are higher in calories and carbohydrates than nonstarchy vegetables. They are considered "carbohydrate foods" in the Diabetes Plate Method. Starchy vegetables have about 80 calories and 15 grams of carbohydrate in a 1/2-cup cooked serving. You want to eat smaller portions of starchy vegetables, fitting them into a quarter of your plate, along with whatever combination of other carbohydrate foods you may choose at the meal.

There are well over 70 different nonstarchy vegetables—lots of options! Here are some examples:

- Asparagus
- Broccoli
- Cabbage
- Carrots
- Cauliflower
- Cucumber
- Eggplant
- Greens
- Green beans
- Lettuce
- Mushrooms
- Okra
- Onion
- Peppers
- Spinach
- Tomatoes
- Vegetable juice

Starchy vegetables include:

- Acorn squash
- Butternut squash
- Corn
- Green peas
- Hominy
- Parsnips
- Plantain
- Potato
- Pumpkin
- Sweet potato

Four things to know about vegetables:

1. **Vary your vegetables.** Eat a variety from all five subgroups: dark green, red and orange, legumes (beans and peas), starchy, and other. Each subgroup contributes a different combination of nutrients, which is why it is important to get a variety.

2. **Enjoy them raw, cooked, fresh, frozen, or canned without added sodium, fat, or sugar.** If you can't find a no-salt-added version of canned vegetables, then rinse and drain them to rinse away about 40% of the sodium.

3. **Keep vegetables healthy by preparing them in healthful ways:** raw, roasted, grilled, microwaved, stir-fried, sautéed, or steamed.

4. **If you currently eat more starchy vegetables than nonstarchy vegetables, try mixing starchy and nonstarchy vegetable(s) together.** It will reduce the carbohydrate if you eat the same portion. For instance, mix sautéed chopped kale with sweet potatoes, or mash steamed cauliflower in with your mashed potatoes.

Eight ways to simplify fitting in more vegetables:

1. **Savor some vegetable soup.** Beyond garden vegetable soup, try tomato soup, pumpkin soup, or roasted caramelized carrot soup. Look for reduced- or low-sodium options. Or make a batch and freeze in microwavable portions.

2. **When dining out, ask for an extra side of vegetables or a side green salad** in place of a potato, rice, or fried side.

3. **Get ahead of the game.** Buy pre-prepped fresh vegetables (many markets sell them packaged, cut up, and ready to cook), or cut up broccoli, cauliflower, and carrots to have on hand to roast, microwave, or mix with a vinaigrette dressing for a salad.

4. **Explore fast ways to cook.** You can't beat the ease of steam-in-the-bag fresh and frozen vegetables. Or you can steam vegetables like asparagus spears, fresh green beans, or bok choy in the microwave. Place them in a microwave-safe dish with a small amount of water, cover, and cook.

5. **Roast vegetables while the rest of the meal is cooking.** Enjoy some now, and eat the rest chilled or reheated for meals later in the week. This vegetable preparation is one of my favorites! See my tried-and-true "formula" to roast vegetables on page 54. It also works on the grill. I place the veggies in a disposable aluminum pan and cook on a hot grill, stirring periodically. Delicious!

6. **Create a DIY (do-it-yourself) superfoods salad bar.** Creating your own salad bar is a simple and great way to fit in more vegetables. (It's a favorite with my family.) See the instructions on page 52.

7. **Pile vegetables on your sandwich.** Whether it is a sandwich or a wrap,

pile on cucumber slices, tomato slices, spinach leaves and/or other greens, onion, bell pepper, or fresh banana pepper or jalapeno pepper slices for a little heat.

8. **Pair vegetables with a yogurt-based dip or hummus.** This combination is a quick and tasty way to fit in a vegetable serving, particularly if you buy ready-to-eat veggies like baby carrots.

How to Make Your Own DIY Superfoods Salad Bar

Would you be more likely to eat a salad if everything was prepped and you had options? One way I've found to make vegetables readily available at home and increase the chance, variety, and amount that my family eats is to create a superfoods do-it-yourself (DIY) "salad bar" right in my own refrigerator. Set aside 15–30 minutes to assemble your "salad bar" for the week. Depending on how many ingredients you decide to include, you may need a little more prep time.

I prep all of the ingredients and store them in inexpensive clear containers that stack, so that it's easy to see what's in them. By stacking the containers, they don't take up too much refrigerator space. I often take some shortcuts like buying carrots or Brussels sprouts already grated or shelf-stable bags of cooked quinoa. You may decide to buy some of the vegetables already prepped and bagged (like fresh broccoli or cauliflower) that you can just transfer into your stackable containers. I then stack everything in one or two 9 × 13 pans, heavy duty foil pans, or baking sheets with sides, along with my family's favorite dressings. Sometimes I put the salad greens in a gallon zip-top bag and lay it on top of the stacked ingredients. I even put ingredients that don't require refrigeration (like nuts, dried fruits, and foil-packed tuna) in the pan, too, so everything is right at their fingertips. Then all they have to do is pull out the pan and pick what they want on their salad that day, and a superfoods salad is ready in moments.

By creating a DIY salad bar in your refrigerator, you can pull together a fast superfoods salad. Superfoods are nutrient-rich foods that offer some important nutrients that can power-pack meals and snacks to enhance your eating pattern and positively affect your health. Keep in mind that there is no single food that holds the key to good health—it's the combination of foods that you portion out on your plate.

On page 53, you will find a number of ingredients you could include as part of your DIY salad bar (and you can certainly add other favorite salad ingredients to the mix). **Superfoods are noted with an asterisk.** The ingredient ideas can be mixed and matched for a variety of flavors, textures, and colors. I enjoy the fresh sweet berries with kale, which is more bitter. While cheese isn't a traditional superfood, a sprinkle of reduced-fat feta or goat cheese adds a savory element and balances the sweet of the fruit. Chewy and tart dried cranberries or cherries, crunchy nuts or seeds, quinoa, mukimame (shelled form of edamame/green soybeans), and foil-packed tuna/salmon add protein and heartiness.

You can use the Diabetes Plate Method when building a salad as well. Even though you're not filling a plate, you can use the same proportions to build a healthy salad: two parts nonstarchy vegetables, one part carbohydrate foods, and one part protein foods.

Superfoods and other DIY salad bar ingredients:

Nonstarchy vegetables

- Broccoli florets*
- Brussels sprouts, shaved/chopped, raw or roasted*
- Carrots, grated
- Cauliflower florets*
- Curly kale, chopped*
- Mushrooms*
- Other salad greens that you prefer, such as spring mix, chopped romaine, or arugula
- Radishes, raw or roasted*
- Red onion, thinly sliced
- Spinach*
- Tomatoes* (cherry or grape means no prepping or chopping)
- Turnips, raw or roasted*

Carbohydrate foods
Starchy vegetables and legumes

- Black beans*
- Frozen peas, thawed*
- Garbanzo beans (chickpeas)*
- Kidney beans*
- Lentils, cooked*

- Mukimame*
- Pinto beans*
- Red beans*

Whole grains

- Cooked bulgur*
- Cooked quinoa (or fully cooked microwavable cups)*
- Cooked wheat berries*
- Corn

Fruits

- Blackberries*
- Blueberries*
- Dried cherries, no sugar added*
- Dried cranberries, reduced sugar*
- Mandarin orange slices, packed in juice
- Pomegranate seeds*
- Raspberries*
- Strawberries*

Protein foods

- Boiled egg (grated, diced, or sliced)*
- Low-fat shredded cheese
- Roasted or grilled chicken, diced
- Roasted turkey, diced or shredded
- Salmon in foil packs*
- Tuna in foil packs*

Healthy fats

- Avocado*
- Nuts: almonds, Brazil nuts, cashews, peanuts, pecans, pistachios, walnuts*
- Seeds: chia, flax, hemp, pumpkin, sunflower*
- Olive oil*

---

*Superfoods.

How to Roast Vegetables

I used to be fearful of roasting vegetables. *Would they turn out right? What if I messed them up?* I've since become a huge fan of roasted vegetables of all types and learned that there's no exact science to roasting vegetables. It's pretty hard to mess them up. There's a multitude of flavor combinations from which to choose. And roasted vegetables are tasty, healthy, and easy! See Table 3.9 for more information on roasting vegetables.

Use this formula when roasting vegetables:

1. **Pick.** Pick your vegetables (about 2 pounds or 8–10 cups). Wash and dry them well (dryness is important so that vegetables roast and not "steam" because of the moisture).

2. **Preheat.** Preheat the oven to 425°F.

3. **Portion.** Portion into 1- to 1 1/2-inch chunks (smaller pieces may take less time to roast, and larger chunks may take more time).

4. **Place.** Place in a 1-gallon zip-top bag.

5. **Drizzle.** Drizzle in 1 1/2–2 tablespoons of olive oil.

6. **Season.** Select your seasonings and add to the bag (or for a "greener" option, use a bowl and tongs).

7. **Shake.** Shake bag and massage vegetables to coat well with oil and seasonings.

8. **Spread out.** Transfer vegetables to a baking sheet lined with a sheet of parchment paper. Spread out in a single layer. This step is important for even roasting. The parchment paper allows for quick cleanup rather than having to scrub the roasting pan.

9. **Roast.** Place tray on an upper (not top) oven rack and roast (25–30 minutes for harder vegetables, 20–25 minutes for softer vegetables) until the edges are lightly browned and vegetables are tender when pierced with a fork.

10. **Stir.** Stir once or twice to allow even browning. Keep an eye on them during the final 5–10 minutes so they don't burn. Depending on the size of the vegetable pieces and the texture you prefer, you may want to roast a few minutes longer or a few minutes less.

More tips on roasting vegetables:

- **To mix vegetables with longer and shorter roasting times,** start vegetables with a longer roasting time in one pan, and then add vegetables with a shorter cooking time to the oven on another pan. When all are roasted, just toss together.

- **Parboil longer-cooking vegetables to speed up roasting time.** Longer-cooking (harder) vegetables, such as potatoes, parsnips, or turnips, can be boiled about 5 minutes to soften and speed up roasting time. Just drain them well and pat dry with paper towel.

- **Enjoying leftovers.** While roasted vegetables are the tastiest hot from the oven, I enjoy leftovers reheated in the microwave, or sometimes taken from the refrigerator and allowed to

TABLE 3.9 VEGETABLE ROASTING TIMES AND SEASONING IDEAS		
Vegetables Requiring Longer Roasting Time (25–30 minutes)	**Vegetables Requiring Shorter Roasting Time (20–25 minutes)**	**Seasoning Ideas**
• Broccoli florets • Brussels sprouts • Butternut squash chunks • Carrots • Cauliflower florets • Parsnips • Potatoes (white, red, yellow, sweet) • Radishes	• Asparagus • Cherry tomatoes • Green beans • Mushrooms • Onions • Peppers (green, orange, red, yellow) • Yellow squash • Zucchini	• Fresh minced garlic or green garlic • Fresh grated ginger • Fresh ground black pepper • Sriracha sauce • Red pepper flakes • Lemon pepper • Coarse sea salt • Low-sodium soy sauce • Basil • Thyme • Parsley • Rosemary • Cinnamon • Nutmeg • Cloves

warm up slightly at room temperature. I also sometimes eat them cold, straight from the refrigerator.

Proteins

Protein foods include a variety of animal and plant sources. Fish, seafood, beef, pork, chicken, turkey, and eggs are examples of animal-based protein foods. They are low in carbohydrate and have a minimal effect on blood glucose. Nuts, seeds, and soy products are plant-based protein foods that are also lower in carbohydrate. Beans and peas (legumes) are high in protein, but they are also higher in carbohydrates. They can be counted as either a carbohydrate food or a protein food. Cheese and cottage cheese are often considered protein foods and dairy servings. For good health, vary your protein routine by including a variety of protein sources. And keep it lean by removing skin or cutting off fat, or by using low-fat cheese or cottage cheese.

Choose Fish and Seafood Twice a Week

Aim to eat fish and seafood in place of meat and poultry twice a week. I encourage you to select a variety, including foods that are higher in heart-healthy omega-3 oils (you'll learn more about omega-3 oils in Chapter 5) and low in mercury, such as trout, salmon, and herring.

A Few Words About Fitting in Nuts and Seeds

- Try a variety of nuts and seeds. Maybe you've only eaten peanuts. Try walnuts, almonds, pistachios, sunflower seeds, flaxseeds, or chia seeds for a change.
- Nuts and seeds are high in calories, so you'll want to eat them in small portions and use them to *replace* other protein foods, not *add* to them. You can fit 1/8–1/4 cup of nuts into your eating plan, but an entire can of nuts can add over 1,000 calories.
- To minimize sodium intake, nuts should be unsalted or lightly salted.

Grains

Grains are a carbohydrate food and can be a good source of fiber and other nutrients. When it comes to grains, the best choices are *whole* grains. Most people don't get enough *whole* grains. They have more nutrients and fiber than processed grains (such as white flour or white rice) and will likely not spike your blood glucose as quickly or as high. Dietary fiber from whole grains may help reduce blood cholesterol levels; may lower risk of heart disease, obesity, and type 2 diabetes; and may help reduce constipation.

Whole grains include the entire grain kernel, while refined grains have been processed, which removes most of the dietary fiber, iron,

and other nutrients. The following are examples of grain foods. **Foods that are whole grain are designated with an asterisk:**

- Whole-grain breads, such as 100% whole-wheat or rye*
- Whole-grain, high-fiber cereal*
- Cooked cereal such as oatmeal*, grits, hominy, or cream of wheat
- Rice, brown rice*, pasta, dal, wheat tortillas, corn tortillas*
- Low-fat crackers, snack chips, light popcorn*, and pretzels

You'll learn much more about whole grains in Chapter 5.

Tips to Transition to Whole Grains: Add Before You Subtract

Used to white bread?
Add in one slice of whole-wheat bread as a swap for one slice of white bread on a sandwich before you take away both slices of white bread.

Used to white rice?
Add some cooked brown rice or quinoa to the white rice to transition your taste buds before you take out all of the white rice.

Fruits

Fruits are a great source of vitamins, minerals, and fiber, making them a healthy choice for people with diabetes. They also contain carbohydrates, so they are considered a "carbohydrate food" in the Diabetes Plate Method. When choosing fruit, focus on whole fruits—they are your best bet. Whole fruits include fresh, canned, and unsweetened frozen varieties. When buying canned or frozen fruit, look for products with no added sugars. Although 100% fruit juice can be part of a healthy eating pattern, fruit juice is much lower in dietary fiber than whole fruit, is less satisfying, rapidly raises blood glucose, and, when consumed in excess, can contribute extra calories. If you choose to include fruit juice, stick to a small serving size of just 4 ounces (1/2 cup).

Watch portion sizes of dried fruit as well—the dehydration process concentrates the sugars in dried fruit, so even a small portion contains a lot of carbohydrate. Look for products with no or limited added sugar, and stick to a small portion size of 2 tablespoons.

If you choose whole fresh fruits that are in season, you can save money and increase variety. For instance, when oranges are in season, you can get variety and increase nutrients by swapping in a blood orange or a Cara Cara orange, for instance.

Tips to help fit fruit into your daily eating:

- **Keep a bowl of fruit on your kitchen table or countertop.** When it's in sight, you get a reminder to fit fruit in.
- **Add fruit to any meal as part of your carbohydrate foods.** At breakfast, add berries to a Greek yogurt. At lunch, top a salad with apple, pear, or mandarin orange slices. At dinner, add peach chunks to a barbecue kabob, or satisfy a sweet craving with sliced strawberries with a drizzle of balsamic vinegar.
- **For fruits that require prep, like melon, cut it up and store in a clear container in the refrigerator** so you can see it to remind you to fit it in.
- **Consider convenience when grocery shopping.** Try pre-prepped packages of fruit, such as pineapple or mango chunks, for a healthy snack in seconds.
- **Make your fruit frosty.** I like to freeze grapes, bite-size banana chunks, and bite-size cantaloupe or honeydew melon chunks and store them in view in zip-top plastic bags for quick, frosty treats.
- **Make small frozen smoothies.** I'm a fan of making a batch of fruit and Greek yogurt smoothies (throwing in some spinach or kale to add a veggie) and freezing them in small jars to pull out and slightly thaw for a snack or as part of a meal.

Dairy

Dairy foods are a great source of calcium, vitamin D, and protein. Milk and yogurt also contain carbohydrates, so they are considered a "carbohydrate food" in the Diabetes Plate Method. Other dairy sources like cheese and cottage cheese are higher in protein and lower in carbohydrate, so they are considered "protein foods." Some dairy foods are also high in saturated fat, such as cheese, full-fat (whole) milk and yogurt, and cream.

Focus on dairy foods that are low-fat and fat-free, such as skim milk, nonfat yogurt, reduced-fat cheese, or fortified soy beverages (commonly known as soymilk). If you're used to 2% or whole milk, making the move to low-fat and fat-free milk can help cut calories and reduce your saturated fat intake. This can be helpful if you are trying to lose weight or if you are concerned about heart disease.

Tip to Transition to Low-Fat Dairy: Add Before You Subtract

I've had many clients transition to low-fat milk by mixing whole milk with 2% milk until they get used to the difference in taste. Then they move to 2% milk. After that, they mix 2% milk with skim milk. Lastly, they move to using straight skim milk (fat-free). It may take some time, but I've seen many successfully make the move. Adding some of the higher-fat milk to the lower-fat milk can help your taste buds transition before you subtract the higher-fat milk altogether.

If you prefer plant-based milk alternatives, soy milk is the closest nutritionally to dairy milk. Other products sold as "milks" made from plants, such as rice, almond, coconut, and hemp "milks," may contain calcium, but are not included in the dairy group because their overall nutrient content is not similar to dairy milk and fortified soy beverages.

The three best dairy/dairy alternative bets:

1. Fat-free or low-fat milk
2. Plain nonfat yogurt, Greek yogurt, or Icelandic yogurt
3. Unsweetened soy milk

Drink Water Instead of Sugary Beverages

Calories and carbohydrate add up quickly when drinking sugary beverages such as regular soda, sweet tea, lemonade, fruit punch, fruit-flavored drinks, sweetened coffee beverages, hot chocolate, and flavored waters (unless they are labeled "zero calorie"). Most people find they'd rather chew their calories than drink them down. Chewing is more satisfying.

With beverages, the goal is to go for drinks that are zero calorie. Water is always the best choice. Other zero-calorie options could include unsweetened tea or coffee (or tea or coffee sweetened with a low-calorie sweetener if you choose), sparkling water or club soda, sugar-free lemonade, sugar-free fruit-flavored drinks, zero-calorie flavored waters, or infused waters. You'll learn how to make infused water in Chapter 4.

Seven tips to help fit in more water:

1. Buy bottled water to easily grab a bottle and know exactly how much you started with and how much you are drinking.
2. Keep a refillable water bottle or travel cup with you to keep water cold and to track how much you're drinking.
3. Use an app to track your water intake.

4. Drink sparkling water or club soda if you prefer carbonation.
5. Add a calorie-free water-enhancer flavoring.
6. Add a twist of lemon, lime, or orange for fresh flavor.
7. Make some creative ice cubes to add to water to give it visual appeal and light flavor. Some favorite combinations are cucumber and basil, cucumber and mint, lime and mint, fresh strawberries, raspberries, or blueberries. Chop the ingredients other than raspberries and blueberries into small pieces and sprinkle into ice trays. Fill with water and freeze.

Healthy Fats

Healthy fats are the "heart-healthy" high-quality fats that come primarily from plant sources. Examples are avocado, olives, flaxseed, pumpkin seed, and sesame seeds. Other examples are nuts such as almonds, Brazil nuts, cashews, hazelnuts, peanuts, pecans, pine nuts, pistachios, and walnuts. The healthy oils are liquid at room temperature and include canola, corn, olive, peanut, safflower, soybean, and sunflower oils (as compared to the unhealthy fats that are solid at room temperature like butter, lard, or shortening). The Mediterranean eating style is rich in heart-healthy, high-quality plant-based fats.

Five simple switches to healthy fat:

1. Switch cooking oils at home. Keep a variety in the pantry and rotate. There are many great flavored olive oils to switch up the flavor in dressings, for dipping and drizzling.
2. Top your morning whole-grain toast with almond butter, cashew butter, or peanut butter rather than butter.
3. Add crunch to a salad with almonds, pecans, pistachios, pumpkin seeds, toasted sesame seeds, or sunflower seeds instead of bacon.
4. Use canola oil or corn oil instead of lard or shortening in cooking.
5. Lightly dip crusty bread in olive oil rather than slathering it with butter.

Partner with a Registered Dietitian Nutritionist (RDN) to Create a Personalized Eating Pattern and Learn to Use the Diabetes Plate Method

Now that you are familiar with the building blocks of foods, the eating patterns that are beneficial in managing diabetes, and how to portion a plate using the Diabetes Plate Method, I encourage you to work collaboratively with an RDN. Together, you can design a personalized eating plan revolving around the pattern that may be most beneficial and doable for you, factoring in personal preferences, needs, and goals. The goal is to find your healthy eating style to maintain for a lifetime. Every change, no matter how small, counts. Small changes add up over time.

Next Steps

1. Identify which eating pattern appeals to you and seems to be a good fit to help you achieve your goals.
2. Identify one change or swap you can make this week to begin embracing that eating pattern.
3. Practice portioning your plate following the Diabetes Plate Method.

Food for Thought

- Carbohydrate is the building block of food and beverages most directly responsible for the rise in blood glucose after eating or drinking.
- There are eight different eating patterns acknowledged to be beneficial in managing type 2 diabetes. Your personal preferences and goals are important considerations when choosing an eating pattern to embrace. Work with your registered dietitian nutritionist to determine which eating pattern is the best for you.
- The Diabetes Plate Method is an easy way to plan and portion meals.
- Small changes add up.
- Find your healthy eating style and maintain it for a lifetime.

CARBOHYDRATES: WHAT THEY ARE, WHERE THEY COME FROM, AND WHY THEY MATTER

Have you heard any of the following advice from well-intentioned family members, friends, or acquaintances?

- "You can't eat sugar or sweets anymore."
- "Avoid bananas and oranges because they'll make your blood glucose levels too high."
- "No more potatoes or carrots for you."
- "Skip the bread and pasta."

The good news is that these recommendations are actually *not true* when it comes to healthy eating with diabetes. Granted, the foods mentioned above are rich in carbohydrate, and, as you may know by now, carbohydrate raises blood glucose levels. But carbohydrate-containing foods do not have to be totally avoided with diabetes. This chapter is designed to bring understanding to what carbohydrate is, what foods and beverages have carbohydrate, why carbohydrate matters so much, and how to manage carbohydrate to, in turn, manage blood glucose. As you read on, you'll learn more about the types of carbohydrate and the importance of quantity and timing. There are many practical illustrations throughout about how to manage carbohydrate.

Carbohydrates: What Are They?

Carbohydrate is one of three key energy-containing nutrients—or building blocks you might say—that make up foods. The other two building blocks are protein and fat. (You'll learn more about protein and fat in

Chapter 5.) Your body needs all three nutrients to be healthy. While carbohydrate, protein, and fat all provide fuel for your body, *carbohydrate is your body's preferred fuel.* It is a ready-to-use source of energy.

Carbohydrate gets the most attention when it comes to diabetes *because carbohydrate is the component of your meals and snacks that is most directly responsible for the rise in blood glucose after eating.* Protein and fat do not affect postprandial (after-eating) blood glucose rise to anywhere near the extent that carbohydrate does, particularly with type 2 diabetes and prediabetes.

The Building Blocks of Food

- Carbohydrate
- Protein
- Fat

Carbohydrate Is Your Body's Preferred Fuel

Carbohydrate-containing foods and beverages = blood glucose rise afterwards

---

There are three main types of carbohydrate:

- Sugars
- Starches
- Fiber

These types of carbohydrate make up the Total Carbohydrate category that you'll see on the Nutrition Facts label on food and beverage packages. You'll learn more in Chapter 6 about using the Nutrition Facts label.

Foods containing carbohydrate have varying amounts of sugars, starches, and fiber and thus have varying effects on blood glucose. In Chapter 6, when we discuss food labels, you'll learn more about how to identify the amount of total carbohydrate in foods and beverages using the Nutrition Facts label, where you'll also see the amount of fiber, total sugars, and added sugars broken down.

Where Does Carbohydrate Come From?

Carbohydrate is found in many of the foods we eat (Table 4.1). And despite what you may hear, many carbohydrate-containing foods are healthy foods. They not only taste good and fuel your body, but also provide important vitamins, minerals, and fiber that your body needs.

What Sections of the Diabetes Plate Method Plate Have Carbohydrate?

- 1/4 plate carbohydrate foods—Yes
- 1/4 plate protein—No (or very little unless protein is plant-based, then Yes)
- 1/2 plate nonstarchy vegetables— Yes, some

TABLE 4.1   WHAT FOODS GROUPS CONTAIN CARBOHYDRATE AND HOW MUCH?

Contain Carbohydrate (raise blood glucose)	Amount of Carbohydrate per Serving (grams)
Starch/grains	15
Fruit	15
Milk/dairy/milk substitutes	12
Nonstarchy vegetables	5
Sweetened beverages	Varies
Sweet treats	Varies
Alcohol	Varies
Do Not Contain Carbohydrate (little impact on blood glucose)	
Meat/proteins	0 (unless plant-based protein, which does have carbohydrate)
Fats	0

Source: Adapted from Academy of Nutrition and Dietetics, American Diabetes Association. *Choose Your Foods: Food Lists for Diabetes.* Chicago, IL, Academy of Nutrition and Dietetics, American Diabetes Association, 2019.

- Glass of milk (if meal plan allows)—Yes
- Side of fruit or other carbohydrate food (if meal plan allows)—Yes
- Add healthy fats—No
- Zero-calorie beverage—No

While some foods, like honey, are pure carbohydrate, many foods contain a combination of carbohydrate, protein, and/or fat. For instance, peanut butter is a mix of all three nutrients. Whole milk, 2% milk, 1% milk, and skim milk have the same amount of carbohydrate and protein, but varying amounts of fat and calories. Chicken is primarily protein with a little fat. However, as you can see in Table 4.2, many foods contain at least some carbohydrate, which means these foods raise blood glucose. *For good health, try to include a variety of nutrient-rich carbohydrate-containing foods at meals and snacks each day, such as dairy, naturally fiber-rich vegetables, fruits, legumes, and whole grains.*

Table 4.3 contains a quiz I often use when leading diabetes programs. You may enjoy checking your carbohydrate knowledge, too! (Spoiler alert: The answers are at the bottom of the table, so cover it before you select your answers.)

Takeaway: Table 4.3 shows that just because a food is "sugar-free" doesn't necessarily mean it is "carbohydrate-free." Many people are surprised when they find out the sugar-free pudding has carbohydrate. The carbohydrate comes from the milk and thickener. However, the sugar-free version does have considerably less carbohydrate than regular pudding.

TABLE 4.2   WHERE CAN YOU FIND CARBOHYDRATE?

All of the following contain carbohydrate in varying amounts:

- Breads and tortillas
- Crackers, chips, and pretzels
- Cereals
- Grains and rice
- Oats
- Beans, lentils, and plant-based proteins (such as soy-based foods)
- Starchy vegetables (such as sweet and white potatoes, corn, peas, and winter squash)
- Fruits and fruit juices
- Yogurt, milk, and milk substitutes (such as soy milk or rice milk)
- Nonstarchy vegetables (such as broccoli, carrots, salad greens, and tomatoes)
- Sweets and desserts (many sugar-free desserts still contain carbohydrate)
- Sweetened beverages (such as sweet tea, lemonade, fruit punch, and sports drinks)
- Other mixed foods (such as soup, chili, and casseroles)

TABLE 4.3   CHECK YOUR CARBOHYDRATE KNOWLEDGE

Which of the following foods contain carbohydrate?

- Baked salmon
- Skim milk
- Fried chicken tenders
- 100% juice apple juice
- Brown rice
- Green beans
- Pizza
- Egg
- Macaroni and cheese
- Carrots
- Banana
- Avocado
- Sugar-free pudding

Answer: All of the foods contain carbohydrate *except* baked salmon, egg, and avocado.

Replace Sugar-Sweetened Beverages with Water as Often as Possible

Whether you have prediabetes or type 2 diabetes, evidence strongly advises avoiding sugar-sweetened beverages (such as sweet tea, lemonade, fruit drinks, and sports drinks) to manage weight and blood glucose and reduce your risk for cardiovascular disease, fatty liver, and tooth decay. Replace sugar-sweetened beverages with water as often as possible. Evidence shows this one switch can reduce the risk of type 2 diabetes by 7–8%. Many people don't realize that consuming sugar-sweetened beverages contributes to a significantly increased risk of type 2 diabetes. If you have prediabetes, studies show that drinking just one sugar-sweetened beverage a day increases the risk of type 2 diabetes (in adults)

Beverage	Sugar in Teaspoons (average)
TABLE 4.4 BUILD AWARENESS ABOUT SUGAR IN BEVERAGES	
12 ounces lemonade	11
12-ounce can of regular soda	10
12 ounces sweet tea	8
12 ounces coconut water	3
12-ounce can of diet soda	0
12 ounces water	0

by 26%. Table 4.4 lists the sugar amounts in popular beverages.

Infused Water: A Flavorful Zero-Calorie Alternative to Help You Drink More Water

There's a multitude of infused water combinations you could enjoy, mixing and matching a variety of fruits and herbs. Come up with your own combinations to suit your taste preferences.

The following are eight favorite flavor combinations:

- Blueberries and orange slices
- Tangerine, lemon, and lime slices
- Lime or orange slices and mint
- Cucumber slices, lime slices, and mint
- Cranberries and orange slices
- Raspberries and lime slices
- Blackberries and sage
- Pineapple chunks and mint

How to make flavor-infused water:

1. Put ingredients in a pitcher or large Mason jar.
2. Fill with ice cubes.
3. Add water to the top. (This also works with unsweetened tea, as another alternative.)
4. Chill in the refrigerator 2–3 hours.

Helpful tips:

- Flavors will intensify the longer your infused water sits, so remove flavoring ingredients when desired flavor is reached.
- Remove flavoring ingredients and discard if water is not all consumed at one time, since these ingredients may become mushy and spoil.
- Store leftover infused water in the refrigerator.
- Try infusing smaller amounts of water on-the-go with an infuser water bottle that has a small center compartment to hold the fruit or other ingredients. This special center compartment will keep ingredients from floating up and blocking the drinking hole.

Sugar Substitutes: At a Glance

What about sugar substitutes? Blue, pink, yellow, green, orange—such is the rainbow of packaging colors for the variety of low-calorie sweeteners available today. Navigating the maze of low-calorie sweetener options can be confusing. The term "sugar substitute" refers to high-intensity sweeteners, artificial sweeteners, nonnutritive sweeteners, and other low-calorie sweeteners. Only a relatively small amount of a low-calorie sweetener is needed because these substitutes are several hundred to several thousand times sweeter than sugar. The U.S. Food and Drug Administration (FDA) has reviewed a number of sugar substitutes for safety and approved them as safe for consumption by the general public, including people with diabetes.

The following low-calorie sweeteners are commonly used as "sugar substitutes" because they are *many times sweeter than sugar,* but contribute few to no calories and carbohydrate when added to foods. They all taste different. If you choose to use a low-calorie sweetener and don't like the taste of the first one you try, switch to another. You may prefer the taste of one over another.

The eight available sugar substitutes in the U.S. (at time of printing):

- Acesulfame-K (brands such as Sunett and Sweet One)
- Advantame (no brand-name products)
- Aspartame (brands such as Nutrasweet, Equal, and Sugar Twin)
- Luo han guo (monk fruit extracts) (brands such as Nectresse, Monk Fruit in the Raw, and PureLo)
- Neotame (brand Newtame)
- Saccharin (brands such as Sweet and Low, Sweet Twin, Sweet'N Low, and Necta Sweet)
- Steviol glycosides (stevia) (brands such as Truvia, PureVia, Enliten)
- Sucralose (brands such as Splenda)

Allulose: A New Low-Calorie Sweetener

You may hear about a low-calorie sweetener called *allulose.* It has the taste, texture, and performance of sugar, but almost no calories. While allulose is not available as a tabletop sweetener (at the time of printing), you may soon see it as an ingredient in many foods and beverages.

Sugar Substitutes: A Personal Preference

When trying to choose the right sugar substitute for you, if you choose to use one, consider the following:

- **Functionality.** *What do you want to use it for? Just to sweeten coffee or tea, or do you plan to cook and bake with it?* Some substitutes perform better in high heat and in cooking and baking.

Learn more about cooking with sugar substitutes in Chapter 11.

- **Taste.** *Do you like the taste?* They all have different flavor profiles.
- **Potential effects.** *Are you concerned about potential effects?* (For instance, individuals with a rare health condition called phenylketonuria [PKU] have a difficult time metabolizing phenylalanine, a component of aspartame.)
- **Cost.** *Does it fit in your budget?* Sugar substitutes are priced at different price points.

Prefer to Stick Closer to Nature?

The two sugar substitutes derived from plant extracts are **luo han guo** (monk fruit extract) and **steviol glycosides** (purified stevia plant extracts). They both have GRAS (generally recognized as safe) status from the FDA.

Summing Up Sugar Substitutes and Beverages

Yes, sugar substitutes can save lots of calories and carbohydrate when swapped in for sugar in beverages like lemonade, soda, and sweet tea. A low-calorie or nonnutritive-sweetened beverage may serve as a short-term replacement strategy for sugar-sweetened beverages,

---

Foods Containing Sugar Substitutes May Still Have Carbohydrate

Let's look at sugar-free, fruit-flavored yogurt: This yogurt contains a low-calorie sweetener but still has 12 grams of carbohydrate per 6-ounce cup, on average. The carbohydrate comes from the milk (from which the yogurt is made) and the fruit.

---

but overall, *the goal is to decrease both sweetened and sugar substitute–sweetened beverages and work on fitting in more water.* Water is the drink of choice.

Sugar Substitutes Takeaway

While replacing sugars with sugar substitutes *could* decrease the intake of carbohydrate and calories (which in turn could benefit blood glucose, weight, lipids, and blood pressure), there's not currently enough evidence to determine whether use leads to long-term reduction in weight, blood glucose, or other factors affecting hearth health (such as lipids and blood pressure). The way to think about it is that using sugar substitutes does not make an unhealthy food choice healthy, but may make it less unhealthy in the sense of saved calories and carbohydrate—as long as you don't compensate with the intake of additional calories (or carbohydrate) from other food or beverage sources.

What Are Sugar Alcohols?

Sugar alcohols are another category of sweeteners that can be used as a substitute for sugar. They have fewer calories than sugar and are not as sweet, so higher amounts are needed to match the sweetness of sugar. Using higher amounts generally brings the calorie content to a similar level as the sugar-sweetened version.

The following are familiar sugar alcohols approved by the FDA for consumption by the general public as well as people with diabetes; however, there is little evidence on benefits. Many of the names, as you see here, end in the letters –ol, as does sugar "alcohol," which can be helpful to quickly spot them on package ingredient lists.

- Erythritol
- Lactitol
- Maltitol
- Mannitol
- Sorbitol
- Xylitol

Sugar alcohols are not generally used in home food preparation, but can be found in many commercial products labeled "sugar-free," including sugar-free chewing gum, candy, ice cream, fruit spreads, mouthwash, toothpaste, and cough lozenges/syrups. If a product is labeled "diet" or "sugar-free," it may contain sugar alcohols. Take note, these "sugar-free" products are not necessarily carbohydrate- and calorie-free! You can quickly check the Nutrition Facts label for any sugar alcohol content. There would be an entry for Sugar Alcohols under Total Carbohydrate. If the product does contain sugar alcohols, you can then scan the ingredient list to see which ones. Learn more about understanding Nutrition Facts package labels in Chapter 6. If you adjust insulin based on carbohydrate consumption, talk with your healthcare team about how to factor in sugar alcohols.

TABLE 4.5   "SUGAR-FREE" ISN'T "CARBOHYDRATE-FREE"

Butterscotch Hard Candy (round disc-shaped)	Carbohydrate (grams)
1 piece regular	4.8
1 piece sugar-free	5.7

Takeaway: Foods labeled "sugar-free" may not be carbohydrate-free. In fact, the total carbohydrate may be the same, or even higher (as you see in Table 4.5). Check blood glucose 1 1/2–2 hours after eating a sugar alcohol–containing food to note the effect.

TABLE 4.6   THE SCOOP ON CHOCOLATE ICE CREAM

Chocolate Ice Cream	Carbohydrate (grams)
1/2 cup regular	18
1/2 cup fat-free, no-sugar-added	26

Takeaway: You might have thought that the no-sugar-added ice cream would be a low-carbohydrate choice. The unexpected carbohydrate comes from sugar alcohols. As Table 4.6 illustrates again, "sugar-free" definitely does not mean "carbohydrate-free." Sugar-free foods can fit in as long as you count the carbohydrate accordingly.

Sugar alcohols do not promote tooth decay and may not cause as sudden of an increase in blood glucose as other sweeteners. However, some people may experience gas, bloating, and gastrointestinal (GI) upset when consuming sugar alcohol–sweetened products. As with sugar substitutes, choosing to use products with sugar alcohols is an individual decision based on your personal preferences and blood glucose goals, and factoring in the potential GI side effects. If you choose to incorporate foods containing sugar alcohols, balance that choice with the potential for GI side effects. As always, your registered dietitian nutritionist (RDN) or diabetes healthcare team can help you decide if including any type of sugar substitutes in your eating plan is the best choice for you.

What About Other "Natural" Sweeteners?

> **Myth or Fact?** "Natural" sweeteners are healthier and don't affect blood glucose as does sugar. MYTH!

There is a common misconception that "natural" sweeteners do not affect blood glucose as much as white sugar. However, these sweeteners *do* have carbohydrate that can raise blood glucose. They *do* have calories. And, thus, they *do* need to be counted in. Here are some examples of natural sweeteners:

- Agave
- Fructose
- Honey
- Maple syrup
- Molasses
- Sugar in the raw

Carbohydrates: Why They Matter

"Managing blood glucose can seem like a balancing act and a rollercoaster ride at times."

Those are words I've heard from patients and clients repeatedly over the years. The truth is, there are over 40 different factors that may affect blood glucose, including food, diabetes medication, activity, biological factors, environmental factors, behavioral factors, and decision-making (see graphic on page 70). Not every person will respond to everything the same way because we're all made differently. And you may respond differently from day to day and over time. The best way to see how different things affect *you* is through personal experience. Check your blood glucose often (or wear a continuous glucose monitor) to look for effects and patterns.

Let's focus just on those factors related to eating for now. As noted earlier in this chapter,

42

Factors *that affect* Blood Glucose

FOOD

- ↑↑ 1 Carbohydrate quantity
- →↑ 2 Carbohydrate type
- →↑ 3 Fat
- →↑ 4 Protein
- →↑ 5 Caffeine
- ↓↑ 6 Alcohol
- ↓↑ 7 Meal timing
- ↑ 8 Dehydration
- ? 9 Personal microbiome

MEDICATION

- →↓ 10 Medication dose
- ↓↑ 11 Medication timing
- ↓↑ 12 Medication interactions
- ↑↑ 13 Steroid administration
- ↑ 14 Niacin (Vitamin B3)

ACTIVITY

- →↓ 15 Light exercise
- ↓↑ 16 High-intensity & moderate exercise
- →↓ 17 Level of fitness/training
- ↓↑ 18 Time of day
- ↓↑ 19 Food and insulin timing

The arrows show the general effect these 42 factors seem to have on blood glucose based on scientific research and/or our experiences at diaTribe. However, not every individual will respond in the same way, so the best way to see how a factor affects you is through your own data: check your blood glucose more often with a meter or wear a CGM and look for patterns.

BIOLOGICAL

- ↑ 20 Too little sleep
- ↑ 21 Stress and illness
- ↓ 22 Recent hypoglycemia
- →↑ 23 During-sleep blood sugars
- ↑ 24 Dawn phenomenon
- ↑ 25 Infusion set issues
- ↑ 26 Scar tissue / lipodystrophy
- ↓↓ 27 Intramuscular insulin delivery
- ↑ 28 Allergies
- ↑ 29 A higher BG level (glucotoxicity)
- ↓↑ 30 Periods (menstruation)
- ↑↑ 31 Puberty
- ↓↑ 32 Celiac disease
- ↑ 33 Smoking

ENVIRONMENTAL

- ↑ 34 Expired insulin
- ↓↑ 35 Inaccurate BG reading
- ↓↑ 36 Outside temperature
- ↑ 37 Sunburn
- ? 38 Altitude

BEHAVIOR & DECISIONS

- ↓ 39 More frequent BG checks
- ↓↑ 40 Default options and choices
- ↓↑ 41 Decision-making biases
- ↓↑ 42 Family and social pressures

diaTribe

Read more about the 42 Factors at **diaTribe.org/42FactorsExplained**
Sign up for diaTribe's updates at **diaTribe.org/Join**

fat and protein may have no effect on blood glucose or may raise it some (particularly in individuals who have type 1 diabetes). Additionally, a high-fat meal may prolong the post-meal glucose elevation resulting from carbohydrate intake. Some people are sensitive to caffeine and see a blood glucose rise after drinking caffeine. And alcohol may raise or lower blood glucose. (You can learn more about that in Chapter 12.) *Without a doubt, carbohydrate affects blood glucose. The three important impactors with carbohydrate, which we'll cover through the remainder of the chapter, are:*

- Carbohydrate type
- Carbohydrate quantity
- Carbohydrate timing

Carbohydrate at Work in Your Body

Simply put, when you eat foods or drink beverages that contain carbohydrate, your body breaks that carbohydrate down into glucose (a type of sugar), which then raises the level of glucose in your blood to fuel your body. Eating too much carbohydrate may raise your blood glucose too high. Eating too little carbohydrate may cause your blood glucose to drop too low, especially if you take diabetes medicines that lower blood glucose. It is important to learn how to manage carbohydrate to achieve blood glucose control. Be prepared for a bit of a balancing act.

Carbohydrate begins to raise blood glucose levels within 15–20 minutes of eating. Maybe you've already noticed that you feel "different" a few minutes after you eat. This feeling may be due to your blood glucose level rising. Before you had diabetes, after eating a meal or snack, your body could sense the glucose coming on board from the carbohydrate you ate and would automatically regulate the amount of glucose in your bloodstream. Now that you have type 2 diabetes (or prediabetes), your body is no longer able to automatically keep the right amount of glucose in your bloodstream, so the more carbohydrate you eat, the higher your blood glucose level may rise (unless you take action to change it). Blood glucose levels peak about 1 1/2–2 hours after you begin eating. After 2 hours, levels should begin to fall off. Managing your carbohydrate intake helps reduce that after-meal blood glucose peak, with the goal of keeping your blood glucose in your target range. *Monitoring carbohydrate intake and noting the blood glucose response are key steps to improving blood glucose after eating. If blood glucose is above target 1 1/2–2 hours after eating, you may be able to bring blood glucose levels into range by reducing carbohydrate.* If you are managing

---

Blood Glucose Targets

Here are general blood glucose targets as recommended by the American Diabetes Association. Talk with your diabetes healthcare team to determine which blood glucose targets are safest for you.

- Before eating: 80–130 mg/dL
- 1–2 hours after the start of the meal: <180 mg/dL

carbohydrate and your blood glucose is still out of range after eating, you may need a diabetes medication added or the amount adjusted if you take one already. Talk to your diabetes healthcare team about this.

Hypoglycemia: What It Is and How to Treat It with Quick-Acting Carbohydrate

"Hypoglycemia" is the medical word for blood glucose that is below 70 mg/dL, which is too low. This condition is a "side effect" or risk of taking many of the diabetes medicines on the market today. If hypoglycemia is not treated, blood glucose may continue to fall to dangerous, life-threatening levels. (For that reason, if you take a diabetes medicine with hypoglycemia as a potential side effect, it's always a good idea to check your blood glucose to make sure it's not low before driving, working on scaffolding, or placing yourself in other situations where your life or the lives of others may be put at risk.) It can be challenging to balance carbohydrate intake (which raises blood glucose) with physical activity and any diabetes medications (which lower blood glucose), along with a variety of other factors that affect blood glucose.

Let's look at an example: If you're going to be doing physical activity—such as spending the afternoon doing yardwork, doing heavy gardening, or working out at the gym—you may need extra carbohydrate to maintain your blood glucose level, especially if you take diabetes medications that may cause hypoglycemia.

Ask your pharmacist about any diabetes medication(s) you take if you are unsure whether these drugs may put you at risk for hypoglycemia. Check your blood glucose frequently—before, during, and after activity and any time that you experience symptoms of hypoglycemia (a list follows). Make sure you are familiar with these symptoms, and always treat hypoglycemia immediately.

Symptoms of Hypoglycemia

- Weakness or fatigue
- Shakiness
- Nervousness or anxiety
- Sweating
- Clamminess
- Irritability or impatience
- Confusion
- Rapid/fast heartbeat
- Lightheadedness or dizziness
- Hunger and nausea
- Sleepiness
- Blurred/impaired vision
- Tingling or numbness in the lips or tongue
- Headaches
- Anger, stubbornness, or sadness
- Lack of coordination
- Seizures
- Loss of consciousness (which can be life-threatening)

What to Do If You Have Hypoglycemia

If you feel like you may be hypoglycemic, check your blood glucose if possible to confirm where it is. For low blood glucose levels in the <70 mg/dL to 54 mg/dL range, use the Rule of 15 to help stabilize your blood glucose.

The Rule of 15:

1. Consume 15–20 grams of quick-acting carbohydrate (see examples that follow).
2. Wait 15 minutes and then recheck your blood glucose.
3. If blood glucose is still under 70 mg/dL, treat with another 15 grams of carbohydrate.
4. Once blood glucose returns to normal (that's >70 mg/dL), eat a meal or snack to prevent reoccurrence.

The following items provide 15–20 grams of quick-acting carbohydrate to treat hypoglycemia:

- Three to four glucose tablets (check package instructions)
- Glucose gel (check package instructions)
- 4 ounces (1/2 cup) fruit juice or regular soda (not diet)
- 1 tablespoon honey, corn syrup, or sugar
- Three round hard candies (such as peppermint or butterscotch discs)
- Smarties candy, jelly beans, or gumdrops (check label on how many to consume for 15–20 grams of carbohydrate)
- 8 ounces nonfat or 1% milk

If you are taking diabetes medications that put you at an increased risk for severe hypoglycemia (blood glucose levels <54 mg/dL), glucagon should be prescribed. Generally, this rule would apply to individuals taking insulin, especially rapid-acting insulin. Glucagon is a hormone that's given by injection or dry nasal spray to rapidly raise blood glucose levels when a person is not able to swallow carbohydrate by mouth. Family, caregivers, and coworkers should know where you keep it and when and how to administer it.

Talk with your diabetes healthcare team about a plan to manage your carbohydrate intake and any diabetes medications to keep your blood glucose from dropping too low, especially during physical activity.

Carbohydrate Impactor #1: Type

All carbohydrate foods do not affect blood glucose the same. Foods containing carbohydrate have varying amounts of sugars, starches, and fiber and thus in turn have varying effects on blood glucose. Some result in an extended rise and slow fall in blood glucose. Others result in a rapid rise in blood glucose followed by a rapid fall. (Learn more about fiber and fiber-rich foods in Chapter 5.)

The type or quality of carbohydrate foods you eat matters. The goal is to choose high-quality foods, which means choosing foods rich in fiber, vitamins, and minerals and low in added sugars, fats, and sodium. Think unrefined, close-to-nature foods. Examples of high-quality carbohydrate foods include vegetables, fruits, whole grains, beans, and low-fat dairy. Try to swap out low-quality carbohydrate foods—foods that are refined, processed, and have added sugars (such as sugar-sweetened beverages and desserts). Small changes add up! By making healthy swaps, you will likely start seeing your blood glucose spending more time in range. The Mediterranean-style and DASH eating patterns in particular revolve around high-quality, unprocessed foods. And certainly the other eating patterns reviewed in Chapter 3 can focus on intentional high-quality choices.

Stick Close to Nature: Choose Whole Foods Over Processed Foods

Let's look at an example: Baked sweet potato versus sweet potato chips. A baked sweet potato with the skin on it is unrefined and "close to nature." It has more fiber and less fat, calories, and salt than processed sweet potato chips.

What About Glycemic Index and Glycemic Load?

You may have read about glycemic index (GI) and glycemic load (GL) or seen an advertisement touting the benefits of low GI/GL foods. Glycemic index and glycemic load rank foods according to their effect on blood glucose and continue to be topics of interest. Research shows that GI and GL in relation to diabetes are complex because blood glucose response to a particular food varies among individuals and

---

Are Sweet Treats Off Limits?

While sweets are not totally off limits, they generally are not considered high-quality carbohydrates. The recommendation is to minimize the consumption of foods with added sugar that have the capacity to displace healthier, more nutrient-dense food choices. The same is true for people with diabetes as for the general public— less sugar is better, and it's particularly important to avoid displacing nutrient-dense foods with empty calories from sweets. This healthy recommendation is for anyone, whether or not they have diabetes or prediabetes.

If you have a sweet tooth, you will most likely find that you can work portion-controlled amounts of sweets into your eating plan. Sweet treats are concentrated in carbohydrate and calories, so you'll want to eat them in moderation and include the carbohydrate in your count (which you'll learn more about later in this chapter). Check your blood glucose 1 1/2–2 hours after eating and note the effect. If your blood glucose is in range, then you made a change for the better!

can be affected by a number of factors. There's no clear-cut answer as to whether GI and GL are of significant help. Evidence currently points to no impact on A1C, with mixed results in regard to impact on fasting blood glucose. Read on to learn a little more about each.

GLYCEMIC INDEX

The GI is a method that ranks carbohydrates on a scale of 0–100 according to how they raise blood glucose after eating. See the glycemic index rankings that follow. Basically, GI predicts the peak blood glucose response.

- **Low-GI foods** produce gradual rises in blood glucose levels because they are slowly digested and absorbed. You may hear these foods called "slow carbs."
- **High-GI foods** are rapidly digested and absorbed and lead to marked elevations in blood glucose.

Two foods having the same carbohydrate content in grams may have differing GI rankings or glycemic loads.

Let's look at an example: jelly beans versus kidney beans

If you have one serving of jelly beans and one serving of kidney beans, and both portions have the same carbohydrate content, the jelly beans will be digested more rapidly and raise blood glucose more than kidney beans. In other words, jelly beans have a higher GI than kidney beans. Of course, to deliver the same carbohydrate amount, the portion sizes of these two foods would be different.

GLYCEMIC INDEX RANKINGS

Understanding glycemic index rankings can seem challenging. Here is a breakdown to help you understand what GI numbers indicate.

- **Low GI:** 55 or less
- **Moderate GI:** 56–69
- **High GI:** 70 or higher

Do you want to know the GI of a favorite food? Check out the online database at www.glycemicindex.com.

If some of your favorite foods have a high GI, you may be able to swap them for lower-GI versions. See Table 4.7 for some examples.

To complicate matters, the GI of a specific food can change based on a number of factors, including the following:

- What else is eaten during the meal or with the food
- How the food is processed and prepared
- Acidity
- Fat content
- Fiber content
- Factors unrelated to the food, including time of day, mealtime blood glucose level, stress, and physical fitness

GLYCEMIC LOAD

"But what about portion size?" you may ask. "What if I'm eating a bite of apple pie, not a whole slice? Does that matter?" The GI of a food does not change whether you eat a bite of apple pie or an entire slice. Eating a larger

TABLE 4.7   SWAP HIGH-GI FOODS FOR LOWER-GI FOODS

High-GI Favorites	Lower-GI Swap
Baked white potato, no skin: 98	Boiled yam, no skin: 35
Pretzels: 83	Popcorn: 55
French bread: 81	Stoneground whole-wheat bread: 59

amount of a carbohydrate-containing food (such as a slice of apple pie) will certainly raise your blood glucose more than eating a smaller amount (a bite of apple pie, for example). That's where glycemic load (GL) comes into the picture. GL takes into account the portion size and potential impact on blood glucose. Substituting low-GL foods for higher-GL foods may modestly improve blood glucose control. A searchable GL database is available at www.glycemicindex.com.

The Takeaway on GI and GL

If you are interested in pursuing the approach of tracking GI and GL, it won't hurt to choose lower-GI and lower-GL foods more often. Swap in lower-GI and lower-GL foods for high-GL foods, when possible, while still being mindful of the portions you eat. Keep in mind that a food's effect on blood glucose may vary from person to person.

Carbohydrate Impactor #2: Quantity

Regardless of which eating pattern you embrace (as reviewed in Chapter 3), managing carbohydrate in some fashion is a priority to help keep blood glucose in range and keep you feeling well. Although there is not a known "perfect" amount of carbohydrate to eat, we do know that the Recommended Dietary Allowance (RDA) for adults with diabetes is 130 grams a day. That amount is determined in part by the brain's glucose requirement to function. Interestingly, the body *can* make enough glucose to meet that requirement, even when a person is following a very-low-carbohydrate eating pattern.

Individualization Is Important: There Are No One-Size-Fits-All Carbohydrate Goals

Having diabetes does *not* mean that you have to totally avoid carbohydrate foods, although many find blood glucose easier to manage and keep in range when eating less carbohydrate. Figuring out how much carbohydrate and which carbohydrate foods to eat are important decisions you'll need to make every day. Through the remainder of this chapter, I'll provide guidance to get you started on managing carbohydrates. I also encourage meeting with an RDN to help personalize these recommendations and provide individualized guidance on optimizing food and beverage choices and meal timing, in coordination with physical activity and any diabetes medication.

Which Is Your Current Scenario?

While managing carbohydrate is a priority, it can be accomplished in several different ways:

- Embracing the Diabetes Plate Method
- Practicing carbohydrate consistency
- Engaging in carbohydrate counting (in some cases factoring in fat and protein)

Often the approach taken to managing carbohydrate is determined by whether or not a person takes any diabetes medication, and, if so, which medication(s). The following recommendations are general guidelines to get you started. Your diabetes healthcare team can give you the best guidance on this. *Which of the following scenarios sounds like you?*

SCENARIO #1: NOT TAKING ANY DIABETES MEDICATION *OR* TAKING DIABETES MEDICATION THAT'S NOT INSULIN.

If this sounds like you, try a simple and effective approach to help achieve blood glucose targets and weight management through an emphasis on portion control and healthy food choices. The **Diabetes Plate Method** can be used for guidance. It shows how to manage calories (by using a 9-inch plate, smaller than many) and managing carbohydrate (by keeping carbohydrate foods to what fits in the 1/4 carbohydrate food section of the plate). The Diabetes Plate Method also emphasizes low-carbohydrate, nonstarchy vegetables. See

Chapter 3 for more information about the Diabetes Plate Method. You may choose to move on to carbohydrate consistency or carbohydrate counting as well.

SCENARIO #2: USING A FIXED INSULIN DOSE(S) EACH DAY OR A SET DOSE OF A DIABETES MEDICINE THAT PRODUCES A RELEASE OF INSULIN INDEPENDENT OF FOOD INTAKE.

If you take a set dose of insulin or medication that produces a release of insulin each day, it may be useful to have a **consistent pattern of carbohydrate intake** with respect to time and amount, considering the insulin action time, to help reach blood glucose goals and reduce the risk of low blood glucose (hypoglycemia). Basically, a fixed or set amount of carbohydrate at each meal/snack accompanies the fixed dose of insulin or medication to help keep blood glucose in range. (That does not mean you have to eat exactly the same foods each day; just eat the same amount of carbohydrate overall.) You may choose to embrace counting grams of carbohydrate or servings of carbohydrate to aid in the consistency. This approach can actually be used by people not taking diabetes medication (or even those with prediabetes) to get in touch with the carbohydrate and amounts in foods and beverages.

SCENARIO #3: USING A FLEXIBLE INSULIN PLAN.

Using a flexible insulin plan allows for greater **variability in carbohydrate intake.** Basically, the mealtime insulin dose is determined by **counting the exact grams of carbohydrate** consumed (and in some cases factoring in fat and protein content) and then adjusting mealtime insulin according to a ratio. That said, many opt to hold their carbohydrate down to keep their insulin dose lower, since more insulin can translate into weight gain. Your diabetes healthcare team can provide guidance on insulin ratios and adjustment.

More About How to Count Carbohydrate

To manage carbohydrate through counting and consistency means tracking the grams of carbohydrate consumed at each meal and snack (whether from food or beverages). While this book focuses primarily on tracking or measuring carbohydrate in grams, you may also track carbohydrate choices (or servings). Here's what that means:

How to Figure Out Carbohydrate Choices

One carbohydrate choice (or serving) = 15 grams of carbohydrate.

To arrive at the number of carbohydrate choices (servings) in a food, take the grams of carbohydrate and divide by 15. So if one serving of a food contains 30 grams of carbohydrate ÷ 15, the result is 2 carbohydrate choices.

Alternatively, to get the number of carbohydrate grams from the carbohydrate choices (servings), take the number of carbohydrate choices and multiply by 15. So if one serving food has 2 carbohydrate choices × 15, the result is 30 grams of carbohydrate.

Whether you choose to manage your carbohydrate intake through counting exact grams, counting carbohydrate choices/servings, or simply by estimating based on experience, use the following three steps to get you on your way.

STEP #1: GET FAMILIAR WITH WHICH FOODS AND BEVERAGES CONTAIN CARBOHYDRATE.

First things first. You have to know which foods and beverages contain carbohydrate before you can work on consistency with your carbohydrate intake. Earlier in this chapter, we took a look at the types of foods that contain carbohydrate and a few examples to get you thinking. Many people have success managing blood glucose by changing the type of carbohydrate foods they eat (where the carbohydrate comes from) and by choosing more healthy carbohydrates (as discussed earlier in this chapter).

There are a number of resources to help you quantify the amount of carbohydrate in foods:

- **Nutrition Facts label on food and beverage packaging**: This is the most direct source for carbohydrate information. (You'll learn lots about how to understand Nutrition Facts labels in Chapter 6.)

- **Reliable online databases.** Two favorites include:
  - CalorieKing at www.calorieking.com. This site is a popular resource that offers a free, expansive, online database that you can search by item or brand and portion size.
  - USDA's FoodData Central at https://fdc.nal.usda.gov
- **Internet search by restaurant for food/beverage names:** Chains and larger establishments often have the nutrition information for their menu items posted online. Many food and beverage manufacturers also post nutrition information for their products on their website.
- **Mobile apps:** There are many free app options. MyFitnessPal is a familiar favorite among my clients.
- **Carbohydrate-counting guidebooks:** Three favorites include:
  - *The Diabetes Carbohydrate & Fat Gram Guide, 5th Edition* (available from the American Diabetes Association at https://shopdiabetes.org)
  - *The Complete Guide to Carb Counting, 4th Edition* (available from the American Diabetes Association at https://shopdiabetes.org)
  - *The CalorieKing Calorie, Fat & Carbohydrate Counter* (updated annually)

Your diabetes care and education specialist or registered dietitian nutritionist may have other suggestions for reputable resources.

Do Chips Have Carbs?

I use this as an example not because I'm advocating to eat chips, but because it's something I often get questions about. Take potato chips or tortilla chips. When checking the Nutrition Facts label, we discover, based on the serving size, that every chip has about 1 gram of carbohydrate. That means if you eat 15 chips, you've eaten 15 grams of carbohydrate. That realization may help you to decide, "Wow, I really need to watch how many I eat!" or "I need to skip the chips."

STEP #2: BUILD AWARENESS OF HOW MUCH CARBOHYDRATE YOU'RE EATING AND DRINKING.

Admittedly, familiarizing yourself with portion sizes and the associated carbohydrate content of foods and beverages takes some thought and effort, especially in the first few weeks. Chapter 7 provides a multitude of tips to size up your portions, both by actually measuring them and by estimation.

To assist in building carbohydrate awareness, you can keep a list of the carbohydrate counts of portions of your favorite foods for quick reference. Some people use a mobile app or the Notes section on their mobile phone. Others prefer a written list or an electronic file. Whatever method works for you is the best method.

Based on years in practice, I find that most people have around 100 foods and beverages that they routinely consume. Because many people eat the same foods from week to week, my clients often share that they quickly become familiar with the carbohydrate amounts in their favorite foods and beverages. Carbohydrate counting becomes much easier with practice. You may find that eventually you can quickly estimate the carbohydrate in food portions based on past experience.

Do Grapes Have Carbs?

Grapes are a close-to-nature, unrefined, high-quality carbohydrate food. And they are much more nutritious than the chips reviewed earlier. But even with grapes, you can get too much of a good thing. Many people are surprised to find that each grape generally has 1 gram of carbohydrate. So if you eat 15–17 grapes, you've consumed 15–17 grams of carbohydrate. Many individuals I've worked with over the years have shared that they could easily eat a cluster of grapes without thinking about it. *How many grapes were eaten? How many carbs came with that?*

Focus on Serving Size and Total Carbohydrate in Nutrition Facts Labels, Not Just Sugar

When reviewing Nutrition Facts labels, focus on Total Carbohydrate for the purposes of carbohydrate counting. Many people tend to focus just on the sugar content of foods, but sugar is only one type of carbohydrate. Looking only at the grams of sugar does not factor in all of the carbohydrate in the food that will affect your blood glucose. Today, begin refocusing your attention on Total Carbohydrate on the Nutrition Facts label to account for all of the carbohydrate in the food or beverage. That's the number to use when tallying your carbohydrate count. See Chapter 6 for more information on using the Nutrition Facts label to guide food choices.

STEP #3: KNOW HOW MUCH CARBOHYDRATE YOU NEED, AND THEN START COUNTING.

Determining the best amount of carbohydrate for you for meals and snacks depends on a number of things, including your:

- Weight
- Height
- Age
- Physical activity

- Food preferences
- Eating patterns
- Diabetes medications (if any)
- Health goals (such as managing blood lipids or weight)

If we consider that the Recommended Dietary Allowance (RDA) for carbohydrate for adults with diabetes is 130 grams a day and spread that out over three meals and a snack, it would translate to around 40 grams of carbohydrate at each meal and one 10- to 15-gram carbohydrate snack. If you're counting choices or servings, that would translate into 2 1/2 carbohydrate choices/ servings for each meal + 1 carbohydrate choice/ serving for one snack.

While that is a very general guideline to cover most basic needs, one size does not fit all. For instance, those who participate in heavy physical activity or work may need more carbohydrate than people who are more sedentary. Men may need more carbohydrate than women. I encourage you to meet with a registered dietitian nutritionist to get personalized carbohydrate goals considering the previously mentioned factors. You may start with a consistent amount at each meal, but find you feel better and blood glucose stays in range with differing amounts of carbohydrate at breakfast, lunch, and dinner. Or you may find you need different amounts on the weekends compared to weekdays. If you lose weight, you may find you need a different amount of carbohydrate. Let your blood glucose be your guide. Note what's working to keep you in range and do more of that.

Basic Carbohydrate Goals for Meals and Snacks

Based on studies, a low-carbohydrate diet is typically a plan that contains less than 45% carbohydrate. And a very-low-carbohydrate diet is typically <26% carbohydrate. Different people need differing amounts of calories depending on whether they're male or female and depending on their height and activity level, among a number of other factors. Table 4.8 shows carb goals for different calorie levels.

Let's look at the 1,800-calorie carbohydrate goals:

If we use 1,800 calories as an example, since it's an average calorie level, and divide the carbohydrate evenly over three meals and one snack for consistency, for both a low-carbohydrate eating approach and a very-low-carbohydrate approach, here's what it would look like:

Low-carbohydrate = 203 grams carbohydrate/day = 63 grams carbohydrate for each of three meals + a 15-gram carbohydrate snack

- So for simplicity, you might go with 60 grams carbohydrate for each meal + 15 grams carbohydrate for one snack.
- If you're counting choices or servings, that would translate into 4 carbohydrate choices/servings for each meal + 1 carbohydrate choice/serving for one snack.
- **This can be a good starting point for many men, or active women.**

TABLE 4.8	CARBOHYDRATE GOALS DEPENDING ON CALORIE LEVEL	
Calories	Goals on a Low-Carbohydrate Diet (g/day)	Goals on a Very-Low-Carbohydrate Diet (g/day)
1,200	135	75
1,500	169	94
1,800	203	113
2,000	225	125
2,500	281	156
3,000	338	188

Very-low-carbohydrate = 113 grams carbohydrate/day = 33 grams carbohydrate for each of three meals + a 15-gram carb snack

- So for simplicity, you might go with 30 grams carbohydrate for each meal + 15 grams carbohydrate for one snack.
- If you're counting choices or servings, that would translate into 2 carbohydrate choices/servings for each meal + 1 carbohydrate choice/serving for one snack.
- A carbohydrate reduction to this level may assist more with weight loss and lowering blood glucose.

Evidence confirms that low-carbohydrate eating results in lower blood glucose and a greater reduction in A1C (estimated average blood glucose). For people with prediabetes, a low-carbohydrate eating plan also shows the potential to improve blood glucose and lipids for up to 1 year. The trick is in maintaining this eating plan, since long-term sustainability can be challenging.

Adopting a very-low-carbohydrate eating plan can initially cause increased urine production and swift reduction in blood glucose. Thus, consult with your diabetes healthcare team before launching into a very-low-carbohydrate approach to head off dehydration, and reduce any diabetes medication doses to head off hypoglycemia. Keep a close watch on your blood glucose, and note effects. If blood glucose is close to or within range, then you know this level of carbohydrate is working. If blood glucose is still above range, you may benefit from further carbohydrate reduction.

Some people notice that meals that are rich in protein and/or fat along with carbohydrate (pizza is one example) lead to a delayed and prolonged rise in blood glucose. Checking blood glucose about 3 hours after eating can help you determine what's going on. Talk to your diabetes healthcare team about what you discover. For people who take insulin, adjustments can often be made in dosing to help counteract this delayed and prolonged rise.

3 Swaps to Reduce Carbohydrate

1. Choose a whole-wheat bagel flat over a whole-wheat bagel. Save over 40 grams of carbohydrate.
2. Choose unsweetened almond milk over dairy milk. Save 10–11 grams of carbohydrate per cup.
3. Choose cooked spaghetti squash or zucchini spirals over spaghetti noodles. Save 35 grams of carbohydrate per cup.

Is It True You Need to Subtract Fiber from the Total Carbohydrate Count?

Have you heard talk about subtracting fiber off the total carbohydrate count to get what some call "net carbs"? Actually, for most people who count carbohydrate, that's not routinely necessary. And it's one more calculation to have to do. Individuals who take mealtime insulin and adjust the dose based on their carbohydrate count may choose to do so when eating foods that contain a lot of fiber.

Managing Carbohydrate Is Like Using a Checking Account

Counting carbohydrate through meal and snack carbohydrate goals is somewhat like using a checking account. At each meal, let's say your goal is 45 grams of carbohydrate. So you have 45 grams in your account to "spend." You can spend these grams on whichever carbohydrate-containing foods you wish. (So while not the healthiest choice, you could even have an occasional splurge, like a chocolate donut, if you plan ahead and allocate grams of carbohydrate to spend on it.) Of course, the goal is to spend the majority of your carbohydrate on a variety of healthy foods. You may find that you end up eating smaller portions of certain foods and eating some foods less often.

If you "overdraw" your carbohydrate account, the "penalty" is that your blood glucose will run higher after the meal. The same rules apply for snacks.

There is no savings account. You use it or lose it at each meal/snack. This approach does not allow reserving or saving carbohydrate from one meal or snack to "spend" on a later meal or snack when you are trying to maintain consistency to level out blood glucose. Spend your carbohydrate wisely to work in those foods that you enjoy!

---

5 Tips To Help Count Carbohydrate In Combination Foods

Foods that contain a combination of ingredients can be tricky to figure out how to count. Examples would be salads, pizza, casseroles, soups, and burritos. Here are five tips to help estimate the carbohydrate count:

1. **Calculate pizza by the crust thickness.** (See comparisons in Chapter 9 on page 164.)
2. **Count salad by the ingredients other than salad greens and veggies.** (See example in Chapter 9 on page 163.)
3. **Count combination entrées by the cup.** For an entrée that has meat/protein and vegetables in a savory sauce, such as stews, soups, and Asian-style dishes, estimate each cup as 15 grams of carbohydrate. For dishes made with rice, pasta, or grains, such as noodle bowls, lasagna, spaghetti with meatballs, chicken and rice, or chili with beans, estimate at 30 grams carbohydrate per cup.
4. **Count the breading on battered or breaded meats.** Estimate 15 grams of carbohydrate for a portion around the size of a crispy chicken sandwich or six chicken nuggets. For larger portions, like a fried pork chop or battered fish fillet, estimate 30 grams of carbohydrate.

Carbohydrate Impactor #3: Timing

Now that we've covered the first two important impactors with carbohydrate—type and quantity—let's turn to the third important impactor: timing. One key thing to remember is, the more consistent your carbohydrate intake is from meal to meal and day to day, the more stable your blood glucose levels are likely to be, particularly your after-meal blood glucose. And in the end, that translates into more in-range blood glucose levels.

If you take diabetes medicine, another key thing to remember is when you need to take your medicine in relation to eating. The action of coordinating medicine and food can help your blood glucose spend more time in range. Keeping your blood glucose levels in range can help you feel better and reduce the risk for problems down the road.

Mexican Meal Carbohydrate Conundrum

Suppose you are eating at a Mexican restaurant and find yourself in this scenario:

You order two beef-and-cheese tacos with a side of refried beans and rice. As you wait for

TABLE 4.9	CARBOHYDRATE COUNTS FOR A MEXICAN MEAL OUT	
Carbohydrate goal: 60 grams for the meal		
Food	Portion	Carbohydrate (grams)
Already eaten:		
Chips and salsa	12 chips + 1/4 cup salsa	20
Margarita	6 ounces	25
Total so far: 45		
Still to come:		
Beef and cheese tacos	2	26
Refried beans	1/2 cup	15
Mexican rice	1/2 cup	25
Total to come: 66		
Grand total: 111		

the food, you munch your way through half a basket of tortilla chips and salsa while sipping on a margarita. After all, it is happy hour! How does the carbohydrate in this meal stack up? Put your carbohydrate-counting skills to work and decide what to do. Table 4.9 helps you sort it all out.

WHAT COULD YOU DO TO KEEP THE CARB COUNT LOWER?

If you eat all of this meal, in addition to the chips and margarita, your carbohydrate intake will total 111 grams—or nearly double your mealtime goal. Oops! Because you've already eaten 45 grams of carbohydrate, you could eat just half of the meal (for 33 grams of carbohydrate) to get a grand total of 78 grams of carbohydrate. Although 78 grams of carbohydrate is above your target of 60 grams, it's much closer to the goal. Or you could eat one of the tacos (for 13 grams of carbohydrate) to get a grand total of 58 grams of carbohydrate, and take the other with the beans and rice home for lunch or dinner tomorrow.

Rate Your Plate

After you create your plate (a 9-inch plate is the perfect size to use), whether you're at a work potluck, church social, restaurant buffet, or in your own kitchen, take a close look at the foods and portions you've put on your plate. Then answer the following questions:

- **Is about 1/4 of your plate filled with a starchy vegetable, grain, or beans?** That's about 30–45 grams of carbohydrate or 2–3 carbohydrate choices.
- **Is about 1/4 of your plate filled with a protein food, such as lean meat, poultry, or fish?** The protein will be carbohydrate-free, unless it's breaded or has a carbohydrate-containing sauce or accompaniment.
- **Is at least 1/2 of your plate filled with nonstarchy vegetables?** That's about 10–15 grams of carbohydrate or about 1 carbohydrate choice.
- **Do you have a serving of fruit and/or a cup of milk or milk substitute on the side to balance your plate (as your carbohydrate goals and eating plan allow)?** The fruit adds 15 grams of carbohydrate or 1 carbohydrate choice. The milk/milk substitute adds another 12 grams of carbohydrate or 1 carbohydrate choice.
- **Is your plate colorful?** (Having a colorful plate helps assure you have a variety of foods.)

The goal is to be able to answer "yes" to all of the questions above. How did your plate stack up? Refer back to Chapter 3 on page 48 for additional guidance on the Diabetes Plate Method. Filling your plate in this manner helps manage carbohydrate and ensure that you're getting variety, a good balance of nutrients, and controlled portions. Small changes add up.

Next Steps

1. Begin compiling a list of favorite foods and carbohydrate counts of portions you frequently eat.
2. Evaluate what you drink and where there's opportunity to fit in more water.
3. Talk with your diabetes healthcare team about the best carbohydrate goal for you, so you can get on your way with counting carbohydrate.
4. Rate your plate using the questions here.

Food for Thought

- Carbohydrate counts most. Carbohydrate in foods and beverages affects your blood glucose levels, so familiarize yourself with the total carbohydrate content of your favorite foods and beverages.
- Reducing carbohydrate (particularly when excessive) helps lower blood glucose.
- Choose carbohydrate foods you enjoy in amounts that fit your carbohydrate goals, so you can feel satisfied.
- Carbohydrate consistency (eating and drinking about the same amount of carbohydrate at meals and snacks each day) helps stabilize blood glucose.
- Balance your plate. When serving your plate, try to keep it colorful, and fill half of the plate with nonstarchy vegetables, one-fourth with lean meat/poultry/fish, and one-fourth with starchy vegetables, grains, or starchy beans. Round it out with a piece of fruit and a cup of milk/milk substitute if it fits within your carbohydrate goals and eating pattern.

OTHER NOTABLE NUTRIENTS

A s emphasized throughout this book, there is no "ideal" eating
pattern for people with diabetes, but rather a variety of eating
patterns that can benefit blood glucose and lower cardiovascular risk
factors. As you step back and evaluate your overall eating patterns, ask
yourself:

Do you steer clear of too much . . .   Do you get enough . . .

- Carbohydrate?   - Lean protein?
- Added sugars?   - Dietary fiber?
- Saturated fat?   - Potassium?
- Trans fat?
- Sodium?

While carbohydrate tends to be of primary focus for people with diabetes because of its direct impact on blood glucose, for general good health,
it's important to routinely take a step back to look at the overall eating
picture. Carbohydrate and its effect on blood glucose was discussed in
depth in Chapter 4. Now let's delve a little deeper into the nutrients with a
specific impact on blood pressure, heart health, and kidney health. In this
chapter, we'll explore:

- Protein
- Fats
- Dietary fiber
- Sodium
- Potassium

Protein

As you may recall from Chapter 3, protein is one of the three building blocks of foods (the other two building blocks are carbohydrate and fat). Protein supplies energy and helps ward off hunger. Protein also helps build, repair, and maintain body tissues. Everybody needs protein to power their bodies, regardless of whether they have diabetes or not.

Which Foods Are Rich in Protein?

Protein is found in many foods. Good protein sources include the following:

- Meat, poultry, and fish
- Eggs
- Milk, cheese, and yogurt
- Soy, beans, and lentils
- Nut butters

Vegetables, cereals, and grain products also contain some protein but in much smaller amounts. An additional consideration with protein foods is that they may contain some fat. The type and amount can vary.

How Much Protein Is Enough?

With the popularity of 10-ounce steaks and three-egg omelets, there is generally no shortage of protein in the average American diet. Most Americans get plenty of protein, but could benefit from more varied protein sources to improve nutrient and health benefits (such as lower-fat sources or sources with healthier fats). Take this into particular consideration if you choose to embrace a low- or very-low-

carbohydrate (and thus higher-protein) eating pattern.

The amount of protein you need depends primarily on your age, sex, and level of physical activity. Generally, 5–6 ounces per day will cover your basic needs. To put that into perspective, the size and thickness of an average

---

Breakfast Protein Power

Find yourself getting hungry mid-morning? Try adding a little protein to your breakfast to hold off hunger.

Here are 7 ways to work protein into breakfast:

1. Boiled egg
2. Scrambled egg whites or egg substitute (such as Egg Beaters)
3. Greek or Icelandic yogurt (richer in protein than traditional yogurt)
4. Peanut butter, almond butter, or another nut butter (some eat it out of the jar with a spoon, while others prefer spreading it on whole-grain toast or apple or pear slices)
5. Low-fat cheese melted on whole-grain toast
6. Almonds or walnuts sprinkled on cereal or yogurt
7. Protein powder or nut butter added to a smoothie

woman's palm is about the size of a 3- to 4-ounce protein serving, whereas the size of the average man's palm is closer to 5–6 ounces. Think back to the 9-inch plate for the Diabetes Plate Method. A portion fitting in 1/4 of the plate for at least two meals a day will most likely have you covered. Your registered dietitian nutritionist can confirm exactly how much protein is best for you and whether you could benefit from a higher-protein, lower-carbohydrate eating pattern to benefit weight or blood glucose.

Did You Know?

- The average woman's palm is about the size of a 3- to 4-ounce serving of meat, poultry, fish, or seafood.
- The average man's palm is about the size of 5- to 6-ounce serving of meat, poultry, fish, or seafood.

---

6 Protein Pointers

1. **Choose lean cuts of meat and poultry.** Lean meat and poultry are more heart-healthy because they have less saturated fat than higher-fat meats. (More information on fats follows later in this chapter.) Aim for 5 grams of fat or less per ounce of protein, and trim away any visible fat. Keep it lean by grilling, baking, or broiling proteins and by using nonstick skillets with cooking spray for "frying."

Words associated with lean cuts of meat include:

- 90% lean (or more)
- Chuck
- Flank
- Loin
- Round
- Tenderloin

2. **Fit in fish at least twice a week.** Many types of fish are rich in heart-healthy omega-3 fats, including halibut, herring, mackerel, salmon, sardines, trout, and tuna. (Omega-3 fats are reviewed later in this chapter on page 95.) Fried fish doesn't count, though! One additional consideration when fitting in fish is mercury: king mackerel, marlin, orange roughy, shark, swordfish, tilefish, ahi tuna, and bigeye tuna all contain high levels of mercury. Excessive amounts of mercury can cause serious health problems. Women who are pregnant or nursing or who plan to become pregnant within 1 year should avoid eating these fish.

3. **Embrace plant-based proteins.** Make beans, lentils, or soy products the focus of your meals. While adding variety, this will also save you money because these protein sources cost less than meat, poultry, and fish. Begin the week with

"meatless Mondays" with a black bean soup for lunch or dinner, for instance. Or opt for a tofu stir-fry or red beans over brown rice.

4. **Nibble on nuts, seeds, and nut butters.** A small handful of almonds, pistachios, soy nuts, or walnuts provides crunch, protein, and heart-healthy fats. Sprinkle a few pine nuts or sunflower seeds on a salad or a few crushed pecans on oatmeal or yogurt. Lightly spread a slice of whole-wheat toast with peanut butter, almond nut butter, or soy nut butter.

5. **Mix in lean, soy-based proteins.** Try soy-based meat alternatives, such as soy-based "bacon," or meatless "beef" or "sausage" crumbles. Snack on soy nuts. Toss tofu or tempeh into soups, casseroles, or stir-fries. Substitute a veggie burger at lunch. Enjoy edamame as a side or snack.

6. **Eggs to the rescue.** As a budget-friendly alternative to meat, switch in an egg. Eat egg yolks and whole eggs in moderation to manage dietary cholesterol intake. Egg whites and yolk-free liquid egg substitutes have no dietary cholesterol and little to no fat, so they are a heart-healthy alternative to whole eggs (1/4 cup of yolk-free liquid egg substitute = 1 whole egg).

Check out the Nutrition Facts label to learn about the fat content of proteins you eat and to look for "hidden" carbohydrate. You'll find these hidden carbs in many plant-based protein sources, such as beans, veggie burgers, or hummus.

Fat

What we're talking about in this section is the fat that you get through what you eat and drink, and the effect that dietary fat ultimately has on

---

Protein Myth Busters

Myth: You should eat protein with carbohydrate (such as peanut butter with crackers) at bedtime to prevent your blood glucose from dropping too low overnight.

Fact: Despite what you may have heard in the past, research shows that protein does not slow the absorption of carbohydrate to prevent hypoglycemia (low blood glucose). In fact, protein *does not* increase blood glucose, but *does* increase insulin response. So the bottom line is that adding protein to carbohydrate **does not help** in treating hypoglycemia or preventing subsequent hypoglycemic episodes.

---

2 Things to Consider When Eating Protein Foods

1. **Generally, protein does not significantly affect blood glucose in people with type 2 diabetes.** However, for individuals using a flexible insulin plan (where mealtime insulin is dosed based on what one eats), considering fat and protein when determining mealtime insulin dosing may help improve blood glucose after eating. If that's you, talk to your diabetes healthcare team about what could work best for you.

2. **Breading, sauces, and gravy may add carbohydrate.** For instance, a plain grilled chicken breast is carbohydrate-free. Basting it well with barbecue sauce adds around 16 carbs.

---

your blood fat levels (which you'll hear called "lipids") and overall health.

Fat is another of the three building blocks that make up foods. All fats are high in calories, containing more than double the calories of carbohydrate or protein on a per-gram basis. Because fats often get a bad rap (particularly in relation to weight and heart health), you may be surprised to learn that fats have important health functions. Some fat is necessary in your diet, and there are actually healthy fats.

The Roles of Fat

Fat in food . . .

- Carries flavor and nutrients
- Gives a smooth and creamy texture (such as in peanut butter)
- Makes foods tender and moist or crispy and brown

Uses of dietary fat in the body . . .

- Carries fat-soluble vitamins so they can be used in your body
- Supplies two fatty acids that your body needs but can't make. These fatty acids are linoleic acid and alpha-linolenic acid.
- Supplies energy in the form of calories
- Helps satisfy hunger by making you feel full

All Fats Are Not Created Equal

Although fat is often referred to in a general sense, there are actually three main types of fat. Each type has different effects, so it's important to know the healthy, high-quality fats from the unhealthy fats and how to swap one for another. Just as choosing high-quality foods is key to healthy eating, so is choosing high-quality fats.

Healthy Fats: Unsaturated Fats

These are the heart-"healthy," high-quality fats that come primarily from plant sources. Think avocado, canola oil, corn oil, olives, olive oil, and peanuts. The Mediterranean eating style is rich in these heart-healthy, high-quality plant-based fats. There are two types of unsaturated fats that are healthy, and you will see these listed on the Nutrition Facts label:

- Monounsaturated fats
- Polyunsaturated fats

Unhealthy Fats: Saturated and Trans Fats

These are the fats that are not healthy for your heart. You will see these broken down and listed on the Nutrition Facts label as well.

Saturated Fats

Saturated fats are solid fats that come primarily from animal sources. Examples are bacon or bacon grease, butter, cream cheese, and lard. Solid fats do to our blood vessels basically what pouring bacon grease down the kitchen sink does to the drain—they clog things up.

Trans Fat

There are two broad types of trans fats found in foods: naturally occurring and artificial. **Naturally occurring trans fats** are produced in the gut of ruminant animals (cattle, sheep, goats, buffalo, deer, elk, and camels). Foods from these animals (such as milk, cheese, butter, and meat products) have naturally occurring trans fat, but they are present in very small amounts. **Artificial trans fats** created in food processing by transforming a liquid vegetable oil into a semi-solid fat (such as stick margarine or shortening) were mostly phased out of the food supply by 1 January 2020.

With type 2 diabetes, eating patterns that are lower in carbohydrate and higher in healthy fat may improve blood glucose, triglycerides, and HDL cholesterol. Swapping in foods rich in unsaturated fat, in place of foods with saturated fat, may additionally improve LDL cholesterol. Hence, if you are embracing a low-carbohydrate, higher-fat eating pattern, incorporating healthy fat sources is important. In general, replacing saturated and trans fat with unsaturated fats reduces total cholesterol and LDL cholesterol and benefits cardiovascular risk (Table 5.1). Small changes really add up.

6 Simple Switches to High-Quality Fat

1. Try almond milk on your morning cereal rather than full-fat dairy milk.
2. Add avocado to a salad or drizzle avocado slices with a splash of balsamic vinegar and olive oil and a sprinkle of sunflower seeds.
3. Mash and spread avocado on a sandwich instead of mayonnaise.

TABLE 5.1   TIPS FOR SWITCHING TO HEALTHY FATS

Choose these . . .		Rather than these . . .	
Monounsaturated Fats	**Polyunsaturated Fats**	**Saturated Fats**	**Trans Fats**
Avocado	Corn oil	Bacon	Vegetable shortening
Canola oil	English walnuts	Butter	Stick margarine
Nuts (almonds, Brazil, macademia, peanuts, pecans, pistachios)	Flaxseed	Coconut milk	
	Pine nuts	Coconut oil	
Nut butters (almond, cashew, peanut)	Pumpkin seeds	Cream	
	Safflower oil	Cream cheese	
Olives	Sesame seeds	Lard	
Olive oil	Soybean oil	Sour cream	
Peanut oil	Sunflower seeds and oil	Shortening	
	Tahini (sesame paste)		

4. Rather than adding butter or bacon drippings to vegetables, try a drizzle of olive oil.
5. Spread on a "buttery" spread containing plant stanols rather than butter (see page 97 for more information on plant stanols).
6. Choose olives over cheese for an evening appetizer.

Takeaway: The quality, or type, of fat you eat is more important than the quantity. To improve the quality of fat that you eat, use unsaturated plant-based fats instead of solid saturated and trans fats when possible.

What About Omega-3 Fat?

Omega-3 fat is a notable type of polyunsaturated fat with heart-healthy benefits. Eating more omega-3 fat may help reduce your risk for heart disease by decreasing total cholesterol and triglycerides. You may be familiar with omega-3 fat as the "fish fat." Many fish (especially fatty fish) are indeed rich in heart-healthy omega-3 fat. So it's recommended to eat fish at least twice a week. (Fried fish does not count!)

Fatty fish rich in omega-3 fats:

- Halibut
- Herring
- Mackerel
- Salmon
- Sardines
- Trout
- Tuna

A Success Story of How to Fit In Fish Twice a Week

One client I worked with was not a huge fish fan, but wanted to try to fit fish in more often. She did not feel confident cooking fish at home. So here was her solution:

- Top a prepared "bag" salad with a foil pack of tuna or salmon at lunch on Monday and Wednesday.
- Make fish her "go to" order when dining out on the weekend. She would occasionally mix it up with tuna or salmon sushi.

Omega-3 fat is not just found in fish. If you are following a plant-based eating pattern, plant sources of omega-3 fat include:

- Chia seeds
- Walnuts
- Flax (ground/milled)
- Soy
- Canola oil

Did You Know?

One ounce of walnuts (about seven whole nuts) meets the daily omega-3 needs.

9 Easy Ways to Work in More Heart-Healthy Omega-3 Fat

1. Top a mini whole-wheat breakfast bagel with fat-free cream cheese and smoked salmon.
2. Add protein to a green salad with foil-packed tuna or salmon.
3. Use dining out as an opportunity to order fish if you don't want to cook fish at home.
4. Munch on a small handful of walnuts for a snack.
5. Sprinkle chopped walnuts over a high-fiber cold cereal or yogurt.
6. Sprinkle ground flaxseed or chia seeds on oatmeal.
7. Stir ground flaxseed into moist, dark dishes such as chili, stew, or meatloaf. My rule of thumb is 1 tablespoon of flaxseed per serving. It's likely that no one will even notice.
8. Grab a handful of soy nuts for a snack.
9. When oil is called for in baking, use canola oil.

While eating foods rich in omega-3s can be beneficial, evidence does not support a beneficial role for the routine use of omega-3 dietary supplements.

What About Cholesterol in Food and Beverages?

The body does not need cholesterol from food to function, since it naturally creates cholesterol. While cholesterol from the diet may raise blood cholesterol, the main culprits in raising blood cholesterol are the saturated and trans fats. More research is needed around the relationship between dietary cholesterol and its impact on blood cholesterol and heart disease in people with diabetes.

Plant Stanols and Sterols: What Are They and Do You Need Them?

Plant stanols and sterols are natural substances found in plant-based foods that may help lower blood cholesterol. They are also called "phytosterols." Sources include fruits, vegetables, vegetable oils, nuts, and seeds.

If you have high blood lipids, you may be able to modestly reduce your total and LDL cholesterol by consuming 1.6–3 grams of plant stanols or sterols per day. Because it's impossible to get enough plant stanols and sterols from natural food sources alone, food companies enrich some food products with these phytosterols. If the package label claims that the food reduces cholesterol, read on and see if the label claims that the food is enriched with plant stanols and sterols.

Phytosterol-enriched foods include select buttery spreads, mayonnaise, dressings, yogurt, milk, fruit juice, cereals, and granola bars. Look for plant stanol/sterol and cholesterol-reduction label claims to help identify these products. Check the label of these phytosterol-enriched products to determine the amount of phytosterols in each serving of the food. The amount varies from one enriched food to the next. Many people choose to incorporate a variety of plant stanol- and sterol-enriched foods to achieve the goal of 1.6–3 grams daily.

Blood Fats (Lipids) Explained: Getting to the Heart of the Matter

If you've had your blood fat (lipid) levels checked recently, you may be trying to make sense of what the numbers mean. To provide perspective, see Table 5.2, which provides an overview of the types of blood fats (lipids) and the general target for each. Talk with your healthcare team about your lipids and what the best targets are for you. If your blood lipids are above target, the type of fat that you eat is extremely important. Swapping healthy fats for unhealthy fats can help keep the heart healthy.

7 Lifestyle Modifications to Help Lower Lipids

If you are trying to lower your lipids, talk with your diabetes healthcare team about the following lifestyle modifications and how to personalize them for you:

1. Adopt the DASH eating pattern.
2. Eat less saturated fat and trans fat.
3. Eat more foods rich in omega-3 fat.
4. Eat more viscous fiber (covered later in this chapter).
5. Include foods rich in plant stanols/sterols.
6. Be more active.
7. Lose weight if overweight/maintain a healthy weight.

TABLE 5.2   BLOOD FAT DESCRIPTIONS AND TARGETS

Type of Fat	Description	Target
Blood lipids	A general term to describe all fats and cholesterol in the blood	Not applicable
Total cholesterol	A waxy, fat-like substance that travels in the blood; includes both HDL and LDL cholesterol The body actually makes most of the cholesterol found in the blood, but some is absorbed from foods.	<200 mg/dL
HDL cholesterol	The "good" or "helpful" cholesterol	>40 mg/dL for men >50 mg/dL for women
LDL cholesterol	The "bad" or "lousy" cholesterol. Too much LDL cholesterol in the blood leaves deposits on blood vessel walls, which can lead to clogged arteries and blood vessels.	Targets vary, factoring in cardiovascular risk. Lower is better. Consult with your healthcare team.
Triglycerides	The most common type of fat in the body; affected by food along with what the body makes	<150 mg/dL

How Much Fat Is Enough?

While there is a definite consensus that high-quality fat should be a priority there is no conclusive "ideal" recommended daily amount of fat. A generally acceptable range for fat intake is 20–35% of total daily calories. So, doing the math, that would mean 45–78 grams of fat per day for an average 2,000 calories. This example gives you some numbers to put things into perspective.

Fat is a significant source of calories (more than double that of carbohydrate or protein). Needs vary from person to person. If you're a runner or otherwise highly active individual, for instance, you need more calories than someone who is sedentary or trying to lose weight, so you could potentially eat more fat (high-quality fat, that is).

Takeaway: Moderation is really the mantra, because all fats are high in calories. Small changes really add up.

How Healthy Fat Calories Add Up: Moderation Is the Mantra

Avocado. Eating avocado is a healthier fat option and is in line with the plant-based and Mediterranean-style diets, but calories can add up quickly. An average avocado runs 250–300 calories.

Peanut butter. Spreading peanut butter on apple slices can be a delicious plant-based or DASH-style snack, but again calories can add up quickly. Spread peanut butter a little more lightly, using 1 tablespoon instead of 2 tablespoons, and you save 100 calories. Or switch to a rehydrated powdered peanut butter (such as PB2) and get 70% fewer calories.

5 Tips to Trim Fat Calories

1. Choose lean cuts of meat and poultry and trim off visible fat. (Refer to the 6 Protein Pointers on page 91 for more protein tips.)

2. Swap in low-fat and fat-free dairy products over full-fat versions.

3. Swap in baked and grilled foods more often for fried foods.

4. Order sauces and dressings on the side when dining out so you can control the amount that goes on your food.

5. Manage portions, since the amount of fat that you eat depends not only on what you eat, but also on how much you eat.

Finding the Facts on Fat

While you're now equipped with a number of tips to improve the quality of the fats you eat, keep in mind that many foods have a combination of these different fats. The more often you emphasize sources that are rich in unsaturated fat over saturated and trans fats,

---

Small Swaps Add Up

Swap 1 cup 1% milk in place of 1 cup 2% milk: **save 20 calories.**

Make this swap twice a day: **save 40 calories.**

Make that twice-daily swap every day for a week: **save 280 calories.**

Make that swap every day for a year: **save 14,560 calories!**

---

the better. Turn to the Nutrition Facts label to familiarize yourself with the amounts and types of fats in a food or beverage. If a label is not available, you can learn about the fat in a food or beverage through reliable, free online databases, Internet searches by brand, or mobile apps. Check out the serving size for the food, too.

Summary: Guidelines on Fat for People with Diabetes

- Focus on making the fat you eat more of the heart-healthy unsaturated fats.
- Eat less saturated fat and trans fat.
- Include more foods rich in omega-3 fat.
- If not following a vegetarian eating pattern, include two or more servings of fish each week.
- Include foods rich in plant stanols/sterols (1.6–3 grams per day is the goal if you have high blood lipids).

Consult with a registered dietitian nutritionist and your diabetes healthcare team for additional guidance and to determine individualized goals for you.

Dietary Fiber

Dietary fiber deserves further mention because it plays an important role in promoting good health. Sometimes referred to as "roughage," dietary fiber is the indigestible portion of plant foods. Fiber is what gives plants shape. Just as fiber provides shape and bulk to plants, fiber bulks up the contents of your intestinal tract. Your body cannot digest or absorb fiber, so instead of being used for energy, fiber passes through your body providing a number of positive health benefits along the way, including the following:

- Aids digestion
- Promotes bowel movement regularity and colon health
- Lowers the risk of some diseases, including heart disease and cancer

Because of these health benefits, fiber-rich eating is encouraged for people with diabetes (as for the general public). The Mediterranean, vegetarian and vegan, and DASH eating patterns in particular (all reviewed in Chapter 3) can help you achieve a fiber-rich diet.

The 2 Types of Fiber: Soluble (Viscous) and Insoluble

Although the focus for many is on getting more fiber in general, the two different types of fiber deserve explanation: soluble fiber (also known as viscous fiber) and insoluble fiber.

Soluble fiber is a type of fiber that dissolves in water (hence the name "soluble"). It then becomes gummy (hence the other name "viscous") and is found in foods such as legumes, barley, oats, and nuts. Think about cooked oatmeal. The gummy residue left in the pan or bowl is from the soluble fiber. Research shows that certain soluble fibers (such as those in oat bran cereal, black beans, and pinto beans) lower blood cholesterol levels and may slightly slow glucose absorption. However, most people consume so little soluble fiber that its effect on blood glucose control is fairly insignificant.

Insoluble fiber, as the name implies, does not dissolve in water. It is found in many plant foods including whole wheat, whole grains, seeds, nuts, brown rice, fruits, vegetables, and root-vegetable skins (such as potato skins). Insoluble fiber absorbs water, bulks up the stool, and sweeps matter through the colon. You may hear insoluble fiber referred to as "nature's broom." Insoluble fiber may help prevent and treat constipation and keep the colon healthy, but it has no effect on blood lipids.

Your best bet is to try to get a combination of both types of fiber by including a variety of whole grains, beans, peas, lentils, vegetables, and fruits in your diet.

How Much Dietary Fiber Do You Need?

Most Americans fall short on the amount of fiber and whole grains in their eating patterns.

Because of the general health benefits of fiber and whole grains, *the recommendation for people with or at risk for type 2 diabetes is to aim for at least half of their grains being whole grains.*

The average American gets around 15 grams of fiber per day, whereas the recommended healthy amount is 14 grams for every 1,000 calories consumed, which means *about 25 grams daily for adult women and 38 grams daily for adult men.*

The good news is that you don't have to eat huge portions of plant foods to get the daily 25–38 grams of fiber! Replacing a morning granola bar with a tasty high-fiber cereal bar (such as Fiber One bars) easily meets up to one-third of your daily fiber goal. Focus on fiber from food sources rather than supplements (because you get coexisting vitamins, minerals, and other plant nutrients). **Choose foods that have >3 grams of dietary fiber per serving,** which means the food is a good source of fiber, according to the Academy of Nutrition and Dietetics and American Diabetes Association booklet *Choose Your Foods: Food Lists for Diabetes.* More is better. **A food that has at least 5 grams of dietary fiber per serving is considered an excellent source of fiber.** Consult with your healthcare team about how much fiber is right for you.

As you've seen, eating patterns rich in fiber have many health benefits. However, to recognize improvement in blood glucose, you would have to eat *a lot* of fiber—more than 50 grams of fiber a day, which isn't realistic for most people. Achieving and maintaining a fiber intake of 50 grams a day can be a challenge, since fiber isn't always palatable; it's hard to consume that amount consistently on a daily basis, and eating large amounts of fiber can bring some uncomfortable intestinal side effects (including gas, bloating, and diarrhea).

How to Get Your Daily Fiber

You don't have to eat huge portions of plant foods to get the daily 25–38 grams of fiber. Here is an example of how you can fit that fiber in through three intentional food choices:

Food	Fiber
1/2 cup raspberries at breakfast	4 grams
1 medium pear at lunch	5 grams
1 cup navy beans at dinner	19 grams
Total	**28 grams**

Whole Grains: Another Way to Get More Fiber

Most Americans are close to the target amounts for total grains, but not enough are **whole** grains, with too many being refined grains. Whole grains are foods containing the entire grain kernel (which means the bran, germ, and endosperm). That means more fiber and nutrients. Choosing whole-grain products in place of refined-grain products is one way to reduce intake of refined grains, while conversely increasing intake of whole grains.

There are many whole-grain foods from which to choose. *Familiar examples* of whole grains include brown rice, oatmeal, popcorn, quinoa, and wild rice. *Less familiar examples* include buckwheat, bulgur, farro, freekeh, millet, and spelt.

Check out the Whole Grains Council website to learn much more about these whole grains and easy ways to enjoy them: https://wholegrainscouncil.org.

What About Fiber-Enriched Products?

Should you include fiber-fortified or -enriched foods to help you reach the fiber goals? While a variety of real close-to-nature food is the first choice, incorporating fiber-enriched foods in place of minimal fiber alternatives can help in upping fiber. While there are mixed opinions, the practical side of me has found that a simple switch such as switching out a breakfast bar for a fiber-enriched bar that easily provides 1/3 of your daily fiber (and easily fits into a carb-managed plan) is a swap in the right direction!

Food manufacturers have begun fiber-fortifying foods such as yogurt, cereals, breads, fruit juices, milk, tortillas, baked goods, supplement bars and beverages, and even ice cream and candies. This fiber can provide health benefits:

- **Bulking fibers** (noted on ingredient lists by names such as carboxymethyl cellulose, methyl-cellulose, or wheat bran) add bulk to the stool and may help reduce constipation while improving digestive health.
- **Viscous fibers** (noted on ingredient lists by names such as agar, guar gum, or pectin) may help lower blood cholesterol and assist with blood glucose control and weight management efforts.
- **Fermentable fibers** (noted on the ingredient lists by names such as inulin, psyllium, or resistant starch) may result in increased mineral absorption, immune support, and insulin sensitivity.

Keep in mind that fiber supplements can interfere with the absorption of certain medications and may reduce blood glucose levels, which could require an adjustment in your diabetes medications.

Your registered dietitian nutritionist (RDN) can recommend ways to increase the amount of high-fiber foods in your meal plan or help you decide if including fiber-fortified foods in your meal plan is the right choice for you.

Quick Tips to Increase Your Fiber Intake

Make at least half of your grains whole grains. Here's an illustration how:

- **Breakfast:** Enjoy steel-cut oats.
- **Lunch:** Choose 100% whole-wheat bread over white or "wheat" bread.
- **Dinner:** Use brown rice or quinoa instead of white rice, or enjoy a whole-grain salad like tabbouleh.
- **Snack:** Munch on popcorn for a snack.

Eat 3–5 cups of fruit and vegetables each day.

- If you fall short on fruits and vegetables, think 25% more. That means if you're eating 2 cups total each day, try adding 1/2 cup more (25%), working toward the goal of 3–5 cups per day.
- Vary your fruit and vegetable choices. Choose them in different colors so you get a good mix of vitamins and minerals.
- Drink 4 ounces (1/2 cup) of low-sodium tomato or vegetable juice for a quick and low-carbohydrate vegetable serving.
- Add fresh berries to your morning yogurt or oatmeal.
- Grill vegetable kabobs as part of a barbecue meal. Favorite grilled vegetables include cherry tomatoes, mushrooms, bell peppers, zucchini, squash, and onion chunks.

Eat fruits and vegetables with the skin on.

- A potato with the skin on has twice the fiber of a peeled potato.

- A 4-ounce apple with the skin on has double the fiber of a carbohydrate-equivalent 1/2-cup portion of unsweetened applesauce.

Eat more legumes (dried beans, peas, and lentils).

- Add garbanzo beans (also known as chickpeas) or kidney beans to a salad.
- Have a cup of black bean, split pea, lentil, or navy bean soup at lunch.
- Spread mashed pinto beans on a whole-wheat tortilla, sprinkle lightly with low-fat cheese, and roll up.

Stick close to nature—the less processed the plant food, the more fiber it contains.

- A whole orange is more filling and has nearly three times more fiber than orange juice.
- Blend fruits and vegetables in a blender rather than "juicing" them. When you "juice," you don't get the fiber that's in the whole fruits and vegetables.

3 Tips to Tolerate Fiber

1. Increase fiber intake slowly to allow your body time to adapt.
2. Drink more water and liquids, because fiber soaks up liquids.
3. Try an enzyme-based dietary supplement designed to reduce gas and bloating (such as Beano).

Sodium

Why the Concern About Sodium?

Too much sodium can lead to significant health problems. One big concern is high blood pressure, which is common among many people with type 2 diabetes. High blood pressure, in turn, may increase your risk for heart disease, stroke, kidney disease, and damage to vision. There is wide agreement in the healthcare world that the average American's sodium intake of 3,500 mg/day is excessive and should be reduced, especially to manage blood pressure. For people with diabetes, as for the general public, the goal is to scale sodium back and *hold your overall daily sodium intake to 2,300 mg or less.* (Significantly lower sodium goals may be considered on an individual basis. However, preference, palatability, and the availability and cost of low-sodium foods are factors that must be considered.)

To put that 2,300-mg goal in perspective, *1 teaspoon of salt contains about 2,300 mg of sodium.* However, one too many shakes from the salt-shaker is not the main source of sodium in Americans' diets. Most sodium consumed in the U.S. comes from salt added during commercial food processing and preparation. Sodium is found in most all food categories. Based on current estimates, almost half of the sodium consumed comes from mixed combination foods including burgers, sandwiches, and tacos; rice, pasta, and grain dishes; pizza; meat, poultry, and seafood dishes; and soups.

Table 5.3 shows how the sodium in processed, canned foods compares to the sodium in fresh and frozen versions.

TABLE 5.3   SODIUM AMOUNTS IN CANNED FOODS VERSUS FRESH OR FROZEN FOODS

Food	Sodium
1/2 cup canned corn, plain	175 mg
1/2 cup frozen corn, plain	1 mg
1/2 cup canned diced tomatoes	130 mg
1/2 cup fresh diced tomatoes	5 mg

Takeaway: Table 5.3 demonstrates that sticking close to nature saves sodium.

You've probably noticed the terms "sodium" and "salt" are often used interchangeably, although here's an important distinction between the two: Sodium is a natural mineral that is also a component of salt (salt = sodium + chloride). Sodium may be naturally present in foods, or sodium may make its way into foods under the guise of "salt." Any way you look at it, less sodium and less salt is the way to go.

Finding Sodium

On food packages, the Nutrition Facts label is the best place to find information about sodium. This information can guide you in making lower-sodium choices.

Although labels may grab your attention with a claim that a food is "low-sodium" or "reduced-sodium," check the exact sodium content on the Nutrition Facts label to see

6 Pointers If Your Blood Pressure Is High (>120/80 mmHg)

1. Decrease sodium toward 2,300 mg/day.
2. If overweight, work on weight loss (even a 5- to 10-pound loss can make an impact).
3. Embrace a DASH-style eating pattern (reviewed in Chapter 3).
4. Moderate alcohol intake (if you choose to drink alcohol).
5. Move more; sit less.
6. Increase potassium intake (unless your healthcare team advises against it because of other health conditions).

TABLE 5.4 SODIUM CONTENT IN SOME FAMILIAR FOODS

Food	Sodium
1/4 cup salsa from a jar	389 mg
3 ounces turkey lunchmeat	660 mg
Two slices of 14-inch thin-crust cheese pizza	760 mg
1 cup canned chunky chicken noodle soup (that's not even half the can!)	850 mg
1 cup low-fat cottage cheese	918 mg
1 tablespoon soy sauce	1,005 mg

how it measures up against your sodium goals. To provide perspective, generally aim for *single servings of a food with <400 mg of sodium and entrées with <800 mg of sodium.*

Foods that are high in sodium may not necessarily taste salty. Check out the sodium contents in the foods in Table 5.4, remembering that <2,300 mg per day is the goal.

Sodium Claims on Labels— Breaking It Down

If you see the following claims on labels, here's what they mean:

- **Salt/sodium-free:** <5 mg of sodium per serving

- **Very-low-sodium:** 35 mg of sodium or less per serving
- **Low-sodium:** 140 mg of sodium or less per serving
- **Reduced sodium:** At least 25% less sodium than in the original product
- **Light in sodium or lightly salted:** At least 50% less sodium than the regular product
- **No-salt-added or unsalted:** No salt added during processing, but the product is not necessarily sodium-free

Do You Savor the Flavor of Salt? Reset Your Salt Preference

The taste for salt is an acquired taste. Just as you can become acclimated to the taste of salty foods, you can "unlearn" that taste preference just as easily—in as little as a week—as I've seen with many of my clients. Over time, the less salt- and sodium-rich foods you eat, the lower your salt threshold or preference will become. You'll be able to taste the salt at lower amounts. For instance, a regular salted-top cracker may taste too salty once you acclimate to lightly salted crackers.

While working toward "resetting" your salt preference or threshold, focus on adding in other flavorful ingredients and begin to appreciate the natural flavor of your food.

I'll never forget hearing a client proclaim, "Wow, I never realized how flavorful green beans are. Now that I've gotten used to less salt, I am appreciating their natural flavor."

7 Simple Steps to Shake Down Sodium

1. **Stick close to nature.** The easiest way to manage sodium is to choose fresh, whole foods that are as close to their natural state as possible. Although small amounts of sodium are naturally present in whole foods, the content is minimal compared with that in processed foods.
2. **Choose no-salt-added** canned goods or plain frozen or steam-in-the-bag vegetables without added sauces.
3. **Omit salt** from the water when cooking pasta and rice.
4. **Rinse and drain canned vegetables and beans** to remove up to 40% of the sodium.
5. **Go for fresh meat when you can.** Fresh foods are generally lower in sodium. Meats and poultry may be brined, so check the Nutrition Facts closely for sodium content. Go for fresh or frozen (not processed) poultry, pork, and lean meat rather than canned, smoked, or processed meats like luncheon meats, sausages, and corned beef.

6. **Consider your condiments.** Sodium in barbecue sauce, ketchup, salad dressing, soy sauce, and many other condiments adds up quickly. Choose "lite" or reduced-sodium soy sauce and no-salt-added ketchup. Add oil and vinegar to a salad rather than bottled salad dressings, and brush meats lightly with barbecue sauce rather than slathering it on.

7. **Only add salt to foods at the table.** By doing this, you'll likely use less salt and will be able to see exactly how much is added to your food (as opposed to when you season as you cook).

Flavor Boosters to Help Reset Salt Preference

- **Herbs** such as green onion, basil, cilantro, parsley, or red pepper flakes (1 tablespoon fresh herbs = 1 teaspoon dried herbs)
- **Aromatics** such as ginger or garlic
- **Vinegars** such as balsamic, red wine, white wine, or rice
- **Citrus juices** such as lemon or lime
- **Strong veggies** such as spinach or kale
- **Mushrooms,** which boost the savory umami flavor
- **Salt-free seasoning blends** such as Mrs. Dash or McCormick Perfect Pinch

<table>
<tr><td>

Considering a Salt Substitute?

If you are considering using a salt substitute, such as "lite" salt, check with your doctor first. Salt substitutes generally contain potassium chloride, which can be a problem for people with certain heart conditions, kidney problems, or people who take certain medications.

</td></tr>
</table>

10 Ways to Cut Back Sodium Without Sacrificing Taste

1. Whisk 1/8 teaspoon of dried thyme or oregano instead of salt into eggs or liquid egg substitute before scrambling.
2. Season mashed potatoes with 1/4 to 1/2 teaspoon each of dried crushed rosemary, garlic powder, and black pepper in place of salt and butter.
3. Use crushed red pepper flakes to turn up the flavor in everything from soups to meats, salads, or even pizza.
4. Forgo the butter, sour cream, and salt on your baked potato, and drizzle instead with 1 teaspoon of olive oil mixed with a sprinkle of fresh chives.
5. Dress up your favorite oil and vinegar dressing with 1/4 to 1/2 teaspoon of dried thyme.
6. Add a splash of flavor, instead of a shake of salt, with balsamic vinegar, white wine vinegar, red wine vinegar, or other flavored vinegar.
7. Finish off asparagus, broccoli, a green salad, or fish with a squeeze of fresh lemon or lime juice and fresh ground pepper.
8. Add a dash of chili powder or smoked paprika to corn instead of salt.
9. Add aromatic ingredients, like onion, green onion, garlic, and ginger, to your dishes.
10. Sample a salt-free herb seasoning blend in place of salt.

3 More Tweaks to Trim Sodium

1. **Add salt at the end of cooking or on the surface of a food (instead of mixing it in).** You'll use less and taste it more.
2. **Use a salt grinder.** Grinding salt is an easy way to add small, controlled amounts. You can even measure with a measuring spoon what each grind yields. Disposable prefilled salt (and pepper) grinders are inexpensive and usually found in the spice section.
3. **Pump up pepper.** Freshly ground black pepper from a grinder has a flavor strikingly different from fine ground black pepper. You'll see that many recipes incorporating black pepper call for fresh or coarse ground pepper for that reason.

Potassium

Potassium Helps Blood Pressure

While the goal is to eat less sodium, the opposite is true for potassium. Eating foods high in potassium can help lower blood pressure by reducing the adverse effects of sodium on blood pressure. In general, adults need around 4,700 mg daily (unless there's a health contraindication). Potassium is often underconsumed.

Choose Potassium-Rich Foods More Often

The DASH style eating pattern emphasizes potassium-rich foods. Bananas are one familiar source of potassium, but there are many more potassium-rich foods. Examples include:

- Apricots
- Beet greens
- Juices (such as carrot, orange, pomegranate, and prune)
- Leafy greens
- Lentils
- Milk
- Nuts
- Potatoes
- Some fish (cod, halibut, salmon, trout, tuna)
- Soybeans
- Spinach
- Sweet potatoes
- Tomatoes and tomato products
- White beans
- Yogurt (nonfat and low-fat)

Food manufacturers may voluntarily list the % Daily Value (%DV) of potassium per serving on the Nutrition Facts label, but they are required to list potassium if a statement is made on the package labeling about its health effects or the amount contained in the food (for example, "high" or "low").

Ways to Increase Potassium Intake

An easy way to bump up potassium is to eat more vegetables, fruits, and legumes. *Here's one way to get half of your daily potassium in one meal that provides 2,351 mg:*

- 3 ounces cooked salmon (534 mg)
- 1 medium sweet potato with skin (542 mg)
- 1/2 medium sliced avocado with 1 cup diced tomato drizzled with olive oil vinaigrette (893 mg)
- 1 cup skim milk (382 mg)

What About Vitamins, Minerals, and Herbal Supplements?

Many people ask about vitamins, minerals, and herbal supplements and wonder if by having diabetes there are any special needs to cover.

- **Routine use.** Routine use of multivitamin or mineral supplements (such as chromium or vitamin D) is not generally recommended without an underlying deficiency.

(continued)

What About Vitamins, Minerals, and Herbal Supplements? (Continued)

- **Metformin and B12.** If you take the diabetes medication metformin, you should get your vitamin B12 level checked at least annually. If the level is low, B12 supplementation is an option then.
- **Magnesium and prevention.** In terms of diabetes prevention, at the time of print, there is some emerging evidence that suggests magnesium supplementation may positively affect blood glucose in people with prediabetes.
- **Herbal supplements.** There's no evidence of blood glucose benefit from routine use of herbal supplements (such as cinnamon or aloe vera). Nutritional supplements and herbal products are not regulated or standardized, so there's concern about adverse effects and drug interactions.
- **Multivitamin.** Talk with your healthcare team about whether you could benefit from a multivitamin based on your health status.

Next Steps

1. Keep a log for 3–4 days of everything that you eat and drink. Using an app such as MyFitnessPal can be particularly helpful. Take inventory of whether you could switch out some foods to improve your fat quality, trim sodium, and boost your fiber.
2. Check the portion sizes of your meat servings. Are they the size of your palm?
3. Did you fit in fish at least once on those 3–4 days you kept the log?

Food for Thought

- Monitor protein portions and keep them close to the size of your palm.
- Choose lean proteins and keep them that way by using low-fat cooking methods.
- Choose heart-healthy monounsaturated and polyunsaturated fats more often, and minimize food sources of saturated fat and trans fats.
- Eat fish more often (at least twice a week).
- Aim to eat 25–38 grams of fiber each day.
- Keep your daily sodium intake at 2,300 mg or less.
- Choose potassium-rich foods more often.

USE FOOD LABELS TO MAKE CHOICES

Would you consider going on a cross-country trip without a navigation app, navigation system, or a map to guide you? Without this important information to keep you on course, you might soon be hopelessly lost.

Likewise in your journey with type 2 diabetes, do you ever find yourself feeling a bit bewildered as you navigate all the food options out there? As you embrace making decisions about food, there's a powerful tool available to you: the **Nutrition Facts label**.

Getting to Know the Nutrition Facts Label

Have you noticed the Nutrition Facts label before? You'll find it on most food and beverages (which are regulated by the U.S. Food and Drug Administration [FDA]). Meat and poultry are regulated by the U.S. Department of Agriculture [USDA], but the required nutrition information is the same as what's on the Nutrition Facts label on other foods. On meat and poultry, you will see nutrient content as packaged but may also see the optional statement of nutrient content as consumed (cooked). As for raw fruits,

Nutrition Facts	
8 servings per container	
Serving Size	**2/3 cup (55g)**
Amount per serving	
Calories	**230**
	% Daily Value*
Total Fat 8g	**10%**
Saturated Fat 1g	**5%**
Trans Fat 0g	
Cholesterol 0mg	**0%**
Sodium 160mg	**7%**
Total Carbohydrate 37g	**13%**
Dietary Fiber 4g	**14%**
Total Sugars 12g	
Includes 10g Added Sugars	**20%**
Protein 3g	
Vitamin D 2mcg	10%
Calcium 260mg	20%
Iron 8mg	45%
Potassium 235mg	6%

*The % Daily Value (DV) tells you how much a nutrient in a serving of food contributes to a daily diet. 2,000 calories a day is used for general nutrition advice.

111

vegetables, and seafood, labeling is voluntary and may be available at the point of purchase. To learn more about foods that may not have labels, check out a free online database like CalorieKing (www.calorieking.com), use a mobile app, or check out one of many guidebooks, such as *The Diabetes Carbohydrate & Fat Gram Guide, 5th Edition,* by Lea Ann Holzmeister, RD, CDE, published by the American Diabetes Association.

The newest version of the Nutrition Facts label was rolled out in 2016 and fully phased in through 2020. It reflects new scientific information, including the link between diet and chronic diseases, such as heart disease and obesity. *The Nutrition Facts label makes it easier to make more informed food and beverage choices. And it is an excellent tool to help build awareness about carbohydrates.*

Because of the overwhelming amount of label information to sift through, I find that people often become confused. In this chapter, you will learn to cut through the confusion and focus on the information you need to know to make the best choices for you.

Top 4 Features on the Nutrition Facts Label to Help You Make Choices

Food labels can help you choose what foods to eat. Say you find yourself standing in the supermarket aisle trying to decide which loaf of bread to buy, with over 20 options on the shelf. Rather than throwing your hands up in frustration and randomly choosing a bread to toss in your cart, take a moment to check out the Nutrition Facts label. What you need to know is how to compare the nutrient numbers and claims of the different breads (and other foods too!).

As you look at the Nutrition Facts, begin to explore the following:

1. How many servings are in the container?
2. What is the serving size?
3. How much Total Carbohydrate is in one serving?
4. How many servings will you eat?

Feature #1: Number of Servings

Check out the number of servings in the package or container. I've been tricked before, thinking that a microwavable cup of black bean soup, for instance, was one single serving. However, I realized, according to the Nutrition Facts label, that seemingly individual container was considered two servings! So it was double the calories and other nutrients I originally thought.

Let's look at popcorn as another example:

The select nutrition information below is from a box of light microwave popcorn.

Servings per bag: about 2
Serving size: about 6.5 cups popped
Calories per serving: 120
Total Carbohydrate: 25 grams

If you pop up a bag of light microwave popcorn, would you eat half a serving (about 3 cups), one serving (6.5 cups), or two servings (the whole bag)?

Takeaway: Compare the number of servings on the label with how many servings you eat. If you eat two servings (which is the entire bag of popcorn), you'll munch down 50 grams of carbohydrate—an entire meal's worth of carbohydrate for many!

Feature #2: Serving Size

The serving size on a food or beverage label is a standardized amount used for comparing similar foods/beverages. You may have noticed that serving sizes have been updated in recent years to be more in line with the amount people actually eat. By law, serving sizes must be based on amounts of foods and beverages that people are actually eating, not on what they should be eating.

Let's look at two examples:

- **Ice cream.** The reference amount used for a serving of ice cream was previously 1/2 cup but is now 2/3 cup.
- **Soda.** The reference amount used for a serving of soda changed from 8 ounces to 12 ounces.

Compare the serving size on the label with the amount you would eat or drink to know the exact amounts of nutrients you'll be getting from that food. There are many mobile apps and free, online food databases that enable you to adjust the serving size of the food of interest to see the associated nutrient content information. Or you can pull out a good old calculator or smartphone calculator to get the job done.

Food Lists: Another Way to Think About Serving Sizes (Calories and Other Nutrients, Too)

You may have heard of what used to be called the "Exchanges" and is now known as "Food Lists for Diabetes." These lists are published by the Academy of Nutrition and Dietetics and the American Diabetes Association in a guidebook called *Choose Your Foods: Food Lists for Diabetes.* The lists provide guidance on serving sizes and can help in meal planning. Like foods are grouped together in similar serving sizes (containing about the same amount of calories, carbohydrate, protein, and fat). There are food lists for carbohydrates and include Starches; Fruits; Milk and Milk Substitutes; Nonstarchy Vegetables; and Sweets, Dessert, and Other Carbohydrates. There are also lists for Proteins, Fats, and Free Foods and guidance on how to factor in Combination Foods, Fast Foods, and Alcohol. The food list serving sizes may be different than the serving sizes on the Nutrition Facts label because they are based on like nutrient content (see Table 6.1 for examples).

TABLE 6.1   TAKE A CLOSER LOOK AT FOOD LIST SERVING SIZES

Food	Nutrition Facts Label Serving Size	Food List Serving Size
Almonds	28 nuts (1 ounce)	6 nuts
Whole-wheat English muffin	1 muffin	1/2 muffin
Raisins	1/4 cup	2 tablespoons
Brown rice	2/3 cup cooked	1/3 cup cooked

Feature #3: Calories

Calories are especially important to factor in when trying to lose weight or maintain healthy weight. And because calories are important, you'll now find them in larger, bolder print on the Nutrition Facts label. Look at the number of calories in each serving. *How many servings do you plan to eat?* If you eat two servings, for instance, then you get twice the calories, too. Checking out calories can also provide perspective in the context of your daily calorie goal.

Let's look at pistachios:
Pistachios are a healthy nut and healthy fat option. However, we can't forget calories. You will be eating 350 calories in a 1/2 cup of pistachios.

Takeaway: If you're trying to lose weight and hold your calories around 1,500 daily, for instance, that 1/2 cup of nuts consumes nearly one-fourth of your daily calories.

Let's consider salsa:
Say you want to use 1/4 cup fresh salsa to top grilled chicken. A 1/4-cup portion of salsa is a "free" food. However, if you desire to use 3/4 cup of salsa to pour over a bean burrito, the larger portion of salsa is not "free" and must be counted.

Takeaway: "Free" doesn't mean "unlimited free." Spread "free" foods out and manage portions.

Are There Really "Free" Foods?

A "free" food is defined as any food or drink with <20 calories and <5 grams of carbohydrate in one serving. A few examples are low-sodium broth or bouillon, 1 tablespoon taco sauce, or lemon juice. **Limit yourself to three servings or less of "free" foods within a day and spread them throughout the day;** otherwise, the carbohydrate in the item may raise your blood glucose.

Feature #4: Total Carbohydrate

When it comes to carbohydrate, this is an important number to know because carbohydrate foods have the greatest impact on blood glucose. (Refer back to Chapter 4 for more about carbohydrate.) Check the grams of Total Carbohydrate in one serving on the Nutrition Facts label. This Total Carbohydrate number does include the grams of Dietary Fiber and Total Sugars (including added sugar), which are indented under the Total Carbohydrate. So you do not need to count those separately or add them to the Total Carbohydrate.

The way I think about it is that total carbohydrate is "one-stop shopping" when it comes to counting carbohydrates. That number is what you'll include in your carbohydrate count if you track carbs. (As an aside, take care *not* to interpret the gram weight of the Serving Size—as denoted alongside the Serving Size on the label—as the grams of carbohydrate. I've found in practice over the years that some people confuse the two.) Compare Total Carbohydrate among items to see what best fits your nutrition needs. Table 6.2 compares two types of cereal—bran flake cereal and frosted flake cereal.

Takeaway: The carbohydrate content of the two flake cereals in Table 6.2 is close, although the Total Carbohydrate in the bran flake cereal is 3 grams less than that of the frosted flake cereal. And the fiber of the bran flakes is 10 times more! That's a big plus! *Which would you choose?* The bran flake cereal would be

TABLE 6.2 COMPARISON OF TWO TYPES OF FLAKE CEREAL		
Nutrition Facts Label Entry	Bran Flake Cereal	Frosted Fake Cereal
Serving Size	1 cup	1 cup
Total Carbohydrate	32 g	35 g
Dietary Fiber	7 g	0.7 g

a healthier option because it has more fiber and slightly less carbohydrate for the same serving size.

Let's look at a 12-ounce can of regular soda: Total Carbohydrate: 40 grams (That's 10 teaspoons of sugar!)

Takeaway: Checking out the Total Carbohydrate helps build carbohydrate awareness. We see that a 12-ounce soda is essentially a whole meal's worth of carbohydrate for many. If you drink soda, there's not many carbs left to eat at the meal. *Could you choose to swap in a zero-calorie drink to save carbohydrate?*

Put the Top 4 Features Into Practice: Let's Look at Canned Black Beans

Start at the top of the Nutrition Facts label:

1. **Look at number of servings per container.** There are 3 servings in the can.
2. **Look at serving size.** The serving size is 1/2 cup beans. If you eat double that

(or 1 cup of beans), you are eating double the calories, carbohydrate, and sodium (and everything else), too.

3. **Look at calories.** There are 105 calories in that 1/2 cup. If you eat double that (or 1 cup beans), you get double the calories, or 210 calories.

4. **Look at Total Carbohydrate.** There are 23 grams of carbohydrate in 1/2 cup. If you eat double that (or 1 cup beans), you get double the carbohydrate, or 46 grams.

Other Label Features That Can Help You Make Choices

Let's now return to the top of the Nutrition Facts label and work our way down, exploring other helpful features on the Nutrition Facts label that can help you make choices.

Feature #5: % Daily Value

I've found that many people are confused by this information. The % Daily Value (or %DV) tells you, for a single serving of that food, how much it contributes of each nutrient toward meeting daily needs for optimum health. While nutrition and calorie needs may vary from person to person, the %DV is based on an average 2,000-calorie-a-day diet to provide a point of comparison. These values can help you understand whether a food/beverage contributes a little or a lot of a particular nutrient to your total daily diet. Trans Fat, Total Sugars, and Protein don't have a %DV listing because no daily reference value has been established for these nutrients.

TIP #1: %DV PROVIDES PERSPECTIVE— 5% OR LESS IS LOW; 20% OR MORE IS HIGH

Let's look at sodium (based on needs for 2,000 calories a day):

- 5% DV or less is low: that would be 120 mg or less of sodium per serving.
- 20% DV or more is high: that would be 480 mg or more of sodium per serving.

TIP #2: %DV CAN HELP YOU TO SEE IF YOU NEED TO RAISE OR LOWER YOUR INTAKE OF PARTICULAR NUTRIENTS

Let's look at fiber and calcium:
The Nutrition Facts label shows a food has a 35% DV of fiber, which makes this food an excellent source of fiber. Then you note the food has 0% DV for calcium, meaning this item is a poor source of calcium. Depending on whether fiber or calcium is a personal health priority, you may decide either to eat or forgo this food.

TIP #3: %DV CAN HELP YOU COMPARE SIMILAR FOODS AND DETERMINE WHICH IS BEST FOR YOU

Let's look at two different cheeses:
What if you're trying to eat heart-healthy and reduce saturated fat, trans fat, and cholesterol intake, but you love a little cheese now and then? Let's compare the %DV of these nutrients in one serving of two different cheeses to determine which will better meet your nutrition goal (Table 6.3).

TABLE 6.3   CHEDDAR CHEESE VERSUS LIGHT CHEDDAR CHEESE

	Cheddar Cheese	Light Cheddar Cheese
Saturated fat	6 g (30% DV)	3 g (16% DV)
Trans fat	0	0
Cholesterol	30 mg (10% DV)	15 mg (15% DV)

Takeaway: Between the cheeses in Table 6.3, the light cheddar would be the better choice because the %DV for saturated fat and cholesterol is lower than the %DV of the regular cheddar cheese.

Feature #6: Fat

As we discussed in Chapter 5, the type of fat you eat is of great importance. The Nutrition Facts label shares the amounts of the following fats:

- Total fat
- Saturated fat
- Trans fat
- Polyunsaturated fat
- Monounsaturated fat

So when you look at the Nutrition Facts label and see that a food has fat, look underneath the Total Fat section and see what types of fat. The goal is to choose foods without trans fat and foods richer in the heart-healthy polyunsaturated and monounsaturated fats. The less saturated fat the better. Dietary cholesterol is less of a focus these days.

Let's take a look at real mayonnaise:
Mayonnaise is a food in which nearly all of the calories come from fat—in comparison to a couple of other creamy sandwich spread options (Table 6.4). *When it comes to fat, by comparison, which of these spreads would you choose?*

TABLE 6.4   COMPARING THE FAT PROFILE IN SANDWICH SPREADS

	Mayonnaise	Extra-Virgin Olive Oil Mayonnaise	Guacamole
Serving size	1 tablespoon	1 tablespoon	1 tablespoon
Total fat	10 g	5 g	3 g
Saturated fat	1.5 g	0.5 g	0
Trans fat	0	0	0

Takeaway: Table 6.4 shows that guacamole has the healthiest fat profile, followed by the mayo made with extra-virgin olive oil (as opposed to regular mayo).

Feature #7: Sodium and Potassium

Give sodium and potassium a little extra attention if you're concerned about high blood pressure. Eating less sodium can help manage blood pressure. And eating more potassium-rich foods may help lower blood pressure and prevent high blood pressure. The recommended intake of potassium for adults is 4,700 mg/day. In general, Americans don't consume enough potassium. (Refer back to Chapter 5 for additional specific guidance.)

Look at the Sodium value to see how the food fits within your daily sodium goal. The recommendation in general is to keep sodium intake to 2,300 mg/day or less. And choose foods richer in potassium (unless your health-care team advises you otherwise).

Tomatoes are rich in potassium, **so, let's look at the sodium in tomatoes:**
- 1/2 cup diced fresh = only 0.5 mg sodium
- 1/2 cup diced can = 130 mg sodium

Takeaway: To get a potassium boost but manage sodium, go for diced fresh tomatoes instead of diced canned tomatoes (or choose no-salt-added canned tomatoes).

Feature #8: Dietary Fiber

Look for foods rich in dietary fiber. Choose foods with >3 grams of dietary fiber per serving, the measure that a food is a good source of fiber, according to the Academy of Nutrition and Dietetics and American Diabetes Association booklet *Choose Your Foods: Food Lists for Diabetes*. More is better. A food that has at least 5 grams of dietary fiber per serving is considered an excellent source of fiber. (Refer back to Chapter 5 for additional detailed guidance on fiber.)

Let's compare the fiber amounts in these soups:
- 1 cup chicken noodle soup = 0.7 g fiber
- 1 cup black bean soup = 8 g fiber

Takeaway: The black bean soup has over 11 times the fiber of chicken noodle soup and is considered an excellent source of fiber.

Look again at the earlier cereal comparison in Feature #4: Total Carbohydrate (page 115) and check out the difference in fiber between bran flake cereal and frosted flake cereal.

Takeaway: The fiber in bran flakes is 10 times that in frosted flakes! So bran flakes would be a much better cereal choice.

Feature #9: Total Sugar and Added Sugars

While the Total Carbohydrate count is your overarching focus for blood glucose control, checking out the Total Sugar and Added Sugars can help you distinguish between sugars that are naturally found in foods/beverages (such as those in fruit/natural fruit juice) and added refined sugars. *Every 4 grams of sugar is equal to 1 teaspoon of sugar!* There's solid evidence linking excessive sugar consumption to an increased risk for heart disease and other illness. The goal is to minimize foods and beverages with added sugars. They don't provide any nutritional benefit.

Remember that the Total Sugars and Added Sugars do not need to be accounted for separately in terms of carbohydrate count.

Let's look at canned sliced peaches:
- 1/2 cup peaches canned in 100% juice = 13 g Total Sugars
- 1/2 cup peaches canned in heavy syrup = 21 g Total Sugars

Takeaway: To conserve carbohydrate and consume less added sugar, choose fruit canned in juice over that canned in syrup.

Feature #10: Protein

There's no ideal amount of protein to eat each day (thus, there is no %DV on the Nutrition Facts label). An average daily amount of protein for people with diabetes (without kidney problems) is typically 1–1.5 grams per kilogram of body weight (a kilogram is 2.2 pounds). If you do the math, for an average 180-pound person, that means he or she may eat 82–123 grams of protein a day. This amount translates into 15–20% of total calorie intake coming from protein. To put that in perspective, every ounce of meat/poultry/fish has 7 grams of protein and every cup of milk has 8 grams of protein. Fruits and fats are the only foods that generally do *not* have protein.

Most Americans get plenty of protein, so actually tracking the amount on the Nutrition Facts label may not be a priority.

Feature #11: Vitamin D and Calcium

In general, Americans don't get enough vitamin D and calcium, which are important for healthy, strong bones, especially in women and older adults. Let the %DV help guide you toward foods richer in vitamin D and calcium. Remember, 20% DV or more is a high %DV.

Feature #12: Iron

As for iron, it's important because your body needs iron to make hemoglobin. Without hemoglobin your red blood cells can't carry oxygen from your lungs to the rest of your body. Again, let the %DV guide you toward foods richer in iron. The goal is 20% DV or higher.

Using the Ingredient List to Make Choices

The ingredient list tells you exactly what's in your food or beverage. Ingredients are listed in descending order by weight. The first ingredient is the main (heaviest) ingredient, followed by ingredients used in lesser amounts. Take, for example, the following ingredient lists from two different steam-in-the-bag broccoli products:

- **Frozen steam-in-the-bag broccoli florets ingredient list:** Broccoli

- **Frozen steam-in-the-bag broccoli with cheese sauce:** Broccoli plus nearly 20 other ingredients

Tip: When looking at ingredients, note whether the food has healthier ingredients (such as whole-wheat flour or canola oil) or less healthy ingredients (such as palm oil, white flour, or high fructose corn syrup).

You can easily spot added sugars as you peruse the ingredient list. **Words that mean "added sugar" include the following:**

- Added sugars (brown, cane, confectioner's, date, invert, powdered, turbinado)
- Agave nectar
- Dextrose
- Fructose
- Honey
- Maltose
- Molasses
- Polydextrose
- Sucrose
- Syrup (corn, maple, agave)

Tip: Choose items without added sugars among the first three ingredients. Compare brands of similar products and choose foods with the least amount of added sugars.

Takeaway: Build awareness of what you're eating. You can make healthier choices just by choosing items that have healthier ingredients listed first in the ingredient list. If you don't recognize multiple ingredients in the item, maybe it's best to put the item back on the shelf.

The more you practice, the faster you will get at reviewing and comparing the Nutrition Facts and ingredient lists. And once you find items and brands that work for you, you may not need to read as many labels and can get your shopping done faster.

To provide a point of reference and get you started on your quest to make good-for-you choices, Table 6.5 gives you some quick tip reminders about the nutrients on a Nutrition Facts label that affect your diabetes.

What About Claims on Labels?

Can you believe claims on labels? Are they true? How can you leverage claims to help guide your choices? As noted earlier in this chapter, the labels on foods and beverages are regulated by the FDA and USDA, which mandate that claims must be truthful to prevent deception. Check out the FDA website (www.fda.gov) for the most current guidelines and definitions of product label claims.

4 Types of Claims That Manufacturers Can Make on Product Labels

#1: Health Claims

Health claims are food label messages that describe the relationship between a food component and a health-related condition (such as sodium and hypertension or calcium and osteoporosis). Health claims are related

TABLE 6.5	NUTRIENT QUICK TIPS
Nutrient	**Quick Tip**
Calories	Guide to calories in a single serving of a food: • 40 calories is low • 100 calories is moderate • 400 or more calories is high
Fats	Lower is better for: • Saturated fat • Trans fat
Sodium	Aim for 2,300 mg/day or less
Total Carbohydrate	Focus on Total Carbohydrate rather than grams of sugars since Total Carbohydrate is what affects your blood glucose most directly. The grams of Total Carbohydrate listed on the Nutrition Facts label already include starch, fiber, sugars, and sugar alcohols—you don't have to count those separately or add those to Total Carbohydrate. If you count carbohydrate choices (servings), approximately 15 grams of Total Carbohydrate = 1 carbohydrate choice (serving).
Dietary Fiber	Foods containing >3 grams of dietary fiber per serving are a significant source of fiber, whereas foods with 5 or more grams of dietary fiber are excellent sources.

to claims about disease risk reduction and cannot be claims about the diagnosis, cure, mitigation, or treatment of disease. There are a number of authorized health claims.

Health claim example for a food low in sodium: "Diets low in sodium may reduce the risk of high blood pressure, a disease associated with many factors."

Of course, if a food features a specific health claim, it must meet strict nutrient content requirements. For a food to sport the low in sodium health claim, it must meet the requirement for a low-sodium food, which is 140 mg or less of sodium per serving.

#2: Qualified Health Claims

Qualified health claims differ from health claims in that they must be accompanied by a disclaimer or otherwise qualified in such a way as to not mislead consumers.

Qualified health claim example for walnuts and heart disease: "Supportive but not conclusive research shows that eating 1.5 ounces per day of walnuts, as part of a low–saturated fat and low-cholesterol diet and not resulting in increased caloric intake, may reduce the risk of coronary heart disease. See nutrition information for fat [and calorie] content."

#3: Nutrient Content Claims

A nutrient content claim is a word or phrase on a food package that makes a comment (directly or by implication) about the nutritional value of the food using terms such as "free," "low," "fresh," "high," and "good source of." Nutrient content claims are strictly defined by regulations and describe the relative amount of a nutrient in a food, without specifying its exact quantity. They give a general idea about the amount of a specific nutrient in a food product. These claims generally appear on the front of food packaging. Nutrition labeling is required for virtually all nutrient content claims.

Nutrient content claim examples: "Low-fat," "high in oat bran," or "contains 100 calories" are examples of nutrient content claims.

#4: Structure/Function Claims

Structure or function claims describe the role of a nutrient or dietary ingredient intended to affect the normal structure or function in humans. Structure and function claims may be used as long as such statements do not claim to diagnose, mitigate, treat, cure, or prevent disease and are not false or misleading.

Structure/function claim examples: "Calcium supports building strong bones," "Fiber maintains bowel regularity," and "Antioxidants maintain cell integrity" are examples of structure/function claim examples.

Are "Natural," "Organic," and "Healthy" Products Better for You?

If the package says a food is "natural," "organic," "vegan," or "protein rich," it has to be good for you, right? Not so fast. These buzzwords abound, and often cause confusion. Yes, some of these products are good for you, and some are less so. Consumers often perceive that "natural" and "organic" imply healthy. But that's not always the case. Just because a food is "natural" or "organic" does not necessarily mean that it's "healthy." Take a closer look at the product and the nutrition information.

Let's look at two examples:

- **Chips.** Although "natural" potato chips might be made with "all-natural" ingredients, they may still be too high in carbohydrate, fat, or sodium to be "healthy" for you.
- **Ice cream.** Although a premium vanilla ice cream could be "natural" or "organic," it's still high in sugar, fat, and saturated fat, so this food would not meet the above criteria for "healthy."

Are "Sugar-Free" or "Fat-Free" Foods Better for You?

When it comes to foods promoted as "sugar-free," people with diabetes should proceed with caution. Many sugar-free, fat-free, or reduced-fat products that are perceived as "diabetes friendly" are in fact made with ingredients that contain carbohydrate (meaning they can raise your blood glucose).

Tip #1: "Sugar-Free" Isn't "Carbohydrate-Free"

Technically, if a food is labeled "sugar-free," it has <0.5 grams of sugar per serving. However, sugar-free foods may still contain carbohydrate, especially if sweeteners such as sugar alcohols (also known as polyols) are used in their preparation. (See Chapter 4 for more information about sugar alcohols.) Sugar alcohols may be listed on the Nutrition Facts label. As a reminder, sugar alcohols do contain calories and carbohydrate, which can boost your blood glucose levels, particularly if you eat a large serving of them. Check your blood glucose after eating them to note their effect on you.

Let's compare two hard candies:
Disclaimer: Let me say up front that I'm not advocating eating candy. However, in my experience, I've found that many people with diabetes suck on hard candy to help with dry mouth—thus the reason for this illustration.

TABLE 6.6 HARD CANDY COMPARISON	
Butterscotch Hard Candy	**Carbohydrate (grams)**
1 piece regular	4.8
1 piece sugar-free	5.7

When comparing the Nutrition Facts labels of a standard product and its sugar-free version, you may be surprised to find that there is little difference in the carbohydrate content (Table 6.6). Or you may find that that the sugar-free variety is actually higher in carbohydrate than the standard version, as is the scenario with the butterscotch hard candy above (the same example we visited in Chapter 4). "Sugar-free" does not necessarily mean "carbohydrate-free." If a product is touted as "sugar-free," check the Nutrition Facts label closely for the Total Carbohydrate content.

Tip #2: Fat-Free Foods Often Contain Carbohydrate

Fat-free foods may initially seem like a great solution to reducing unhealthy fat. However, many of today's fat replacers in foods are carbohydrate-based. Although the fat content in a product might be lower, the carbohydrate content can be higher and thus affect your blood glucose. Table 6.7 gives nutritional information for two types of ranch-style dressing.

TABLE 6.7   COMPARISON OF REGULAR AND FAT-FREE RANCH DRESSING

Food	Calories	Fat (grams)	Carbohydrate (grams)
2 tablespoons regular ranch-style salad dressing	140	14	2
2 tablespoons fat-free ranch-style salad dressing	30	0	6

Takeaway: After reading the Nutrition Facts label and finding that the fat-free version of ranch salad dressing contains a significant amount of carbohydrate, you may decide to eat a small portion of the "real thing."

Let's look at ice cream:

That name-brand low-fat, no-sugar-added vanilla ice cream sandwich has 29 grams of carbohydrate; the same name-brand low-fat regular version of that vanilla ice cream sandwich has 30 grams of fat.

Which one would you choose? Your taste buds may tell you to go with the regular low-fat version (which generally will cost less than the sugar-free version, too). In this case, follow your taste buds and go with the regular version over the sugar-free version, since the carbohydrate is about the same.

Gluten Guidance

What Is Gluten?

Gluten is a protein in barley, rye, and wheat. Gluten is also found in crossbred hybrid grains such as triticale, which is a cross between wheat and rye. People who don't eat gluten also need to be cautious with oats; while oats do not innately have gluten, they may come into contact with gluten during processing. If gluten is a concern for you, do not eat oats unless they are labeled "gluten-free."

Knowing about gluten is of utmost importance for those living with gluten sensitivity, or celiac disease. You may have heard of the higher prevalence of celiac disease among people living with type 1 diabetes in particular.

For People with Celiac Disease

In people with celiac disease, eating gluten triggers the production of antibodies that attack and damage the lining of the small intestine, leading to an array of uncomfortable symptoms. Such damage limits the ability of the small intestine to absorb nutrients and increases the risk for other serious health problems, including nutritional deficiencies (such as vitamin D deficiency), osteoporosis, growth retardation, infertility, miscarriages, short stature, and intestinal cancers. The only way to manage celiac disease is to completely avoid all foods that contain gluten. Following a gluten-free lifestyle helps prevent permanent damage to the body and helps those with celiac disease feel better.

For People with Gluten Sensitivity

People with gluten sensitivity also experience uncomfortable symptoms when consuming items with gluten; however, they test negative for celiac disease, and actual damage to their intestine does not occur. Avoiding foods with gluten also helps relieve symptoms for people with gluten sensitivity. The number of people who choose a gluten-free lifestyle is on the rise.

If you cannot tolerate gluten, read labels carefully. Labeling standards are in place to ensure that items labeled "gluten-free" meet a standard for gluten content, thus instilling confidence that "gluten-free" items are safe for consumption.

"Gluten-Free" by Definition

According to the FDA, foods labeled "gluten-free" are either inherently free of gluten or do not contain an ingredient that is:

- A gluten-containing grain (e.g., spelt wheat);
- Derived from a gluten-containing grain that has not been processed to remove gluten (e.g., wheat flour); *or*

- Derived from a gluten-containing grain that has been processed to remove gluten (e.g., wheat starch).

Any unavoidable presence of gluten in the food must be less than 20 parts per million. Restaurants and other establishments making a gluten-free claim on their menus should be consistent with the FDA's definition.

If celiac disease or gluten intolerance is a concern for you, talk with your registered dietitian nutritionist (RDN) or doctor for further guidance on gluten-free eating.

Using the Nutrition Facts Label to Make Food Choices That Follow Your Eating Plan

Using the Nutrition Facts label can help you discover many healthy swaps to align with the eating pattern you are embracing. Table 6.8 shows a few discoveries made when using the Nutrition Facts label to help choose foods.

Discovery that comes from building awareness through using food labels can drive positive behavior change. Allow some time up front to get familiar with food labels. Maybe start by checking out labels on items in your kitchen or refrigerator. Over time, once you've identified the best choices for you, future shopping trips will go faster. Periodically, do a checkup on labels to catch any changes in ingredients and numbers. The time you spend now will save you time—and protect your health—for years into the future.

TABLE 6.8   DISCOVERIES MADE BY USING THE NUTRITION FACTS LABEL TO GUIDE FOOD CHOICES

Eating Pattern	Choose this . . .	Instead of this . . .	And you get . . .
Mediterranean-style	Olive oil–based vinaigrette	Creamy salad dressing	Healthier fats
DASH style	Whole-grain bread	White bread	Whole grains and more fiber
Plant-based	Unsweetened almond milk	Unsweetened soy milk	Less calories and carbohydrate
Low-carbohydrate	Light cheddar cheese	Regular cheddar cheese	Less fat and calories
Paleo	Wild-caught tuna canned in water	Wild-caught tuna canned in oil	Less fat and calories
Low-fat	Oatmeal	Cream of wheat	More fiber

Next Steps

Put your label-reading skills to the test by doing a bit of shelf searching. Find three foods or beverages in your refrigerator or kitchen shelves and practice:

1. Check the number of servings in the container. *Is that a surprise or not?*
2. Check the serving size. *Is that the serving you typically eat?*
3. Check the calories in one serving. *Is a serving of that food worth the calories?*
4. Check the Total Carbohydrate. *Would a serving fit in your carbohydrate goal for a meal or snack? Is the carbohydrate worth it?*

Food for Thought

- The Nutrition Facts label makes it easier to make more informed food and beverage choices and can help build carbohydrate awareness.
- Get familiar first with servings per container and serving size, and then check total calories and Total Carbohydrate in a serving.

- Label claims can help direct you toward foods that may work for you.
- Check out the ingredient list looking specifically for familiar healthy ingredients. Often the shorter the ingredient list, the better.
- Feel overwhelmed by the nutrition information label? Get back to basics and focus on serving size and amount of Total Carbohydrate.

MANAGE YOUR PORTIONS

How Important Are Portion Sizes?

Managing portions is a big concern because larger portions mean more calories, which can translate into extra weight. And managing weight is a priority for many people with or at risk for type 2 diabetes.

Because extra body fat is linked to insulin resistance, and thus challenges with managing blood glucose, weight loss has long been a recommended strategy for overweight or obese adults with or at risk for diabetes. Prevention of weight gain is equally important.

Larger portions also often mean more carbohydrate (and likely more fat and sodium, too) and thus a greater impact on blood glucose levels.

Ask Yourself: Are the Calories and Carbohydrate Worth It?

When discussing portions and food choices with my clients, I often challenge them to ask themselves a question if considering whether or not to eat a particular food: *Are the calories and carbohydrate worth it?* Sometimes the answer was "yes," but more often than not, the answer was "no." **Here are three scenarios to consider to get you thinking:**

1. When eating out, is ordering a "value meal" or going to an "all-you-can-eat" buffet really a bargain if you eat excessive calories and your blood glucose is above target 2 hours later because of larger portions of carbohydrate foods?

(continued)

Ask Yourself: Are the Calories and Carbohydrate Worth It? (Continued)

2. Is a slice of apple pie worth it, if you had to dance energetically for 40 minutes to burn off the calories?*

3. Is the extra 1-ounce cube of cheese at the party worth it, if you had to cycle about 10 minutes to burn off the extra calories?*

*These calculations are based on averages for a 150-pound woman.

Portion Distortion: Have You Experienced It?

Have you ever found yourself thinking, "I can't believe I ate the whole thing!"? It's no secret that portion sizes in the U.S. have inflated over the years. Food portions are larger than they were 25 years ago at almost every food venue, from markets to vending machines to restaurants.

Consider around 25 years ago . . .

*   *Then* a bagel was 3 inches in diameter and 140 calories. *Now* the average bagel is 5–6 inches in diameter and 350 calories. An average 5'10" man weighing about 155 pounds would have to play basketball for 30 minutes to burn off the extra 210 calories!

*   *Then* a standard serving of French fries was 2.4 ounces and 210 calories. *Now* the serving size is nearly double that, at about 5 ounces and 410 calories. That same average 5'10" man weighing about 155 pounds would have to do 75 minutes of light yard work to burn off those 410 calories!

Consumer perceptions of appropriate portion sizes have become distorted, with larger portions now viewed as the normal amount to eat on a single occasion.

Ways to Build Awareness of Portion Sizes

Portion Size Tip #1: Read Nutrition Information

A positive trend is the increasing availability of nutrition information—from the Nutrition Facts label on food packages to calorie content and other nutrition information at a restaurant—that raises consumer awareness and enables you to make informed decisions. You can compare the portion you actually eat to the serving size in the nutrition information. If you eat double the serving size noted, then double the calorie, carbohydrate, and other nutrient counts, too.

Portion Size Tip #2: Choose Dish and Glass Size Wisely

Just as portion sizes have increased, so have the sizes of dishes and glasses. Because a "normal"-size portion looks small in a large

Let's Practice: Whole-Grain Wheat Square Cereal (such as Wheat Chex)

Let's say you decide to have a whole-grain wheat square cereal for breakfast. Here's what you see for the nutrition information:

Serving size: 3/4 cup
Calories: 150
Fat: 1 g
Sodium: 270 mg
Total Carbohydrate: 39 g

But you know that you typically eat more cereal than that. If you *choose to eat 1 1/2 cups*, which is double the serving size, that means double the calories, fat, sodium, and carbohydrate. So here's what you would get:

Serving size: 1 1/2 cups (3/4 cup × 2)
Calories: 300 calories (150 calories × 2)
Fat: 2 g (1 g × 2)
Sodium: 540 mg (270 mg × 2)
Total Carbohydrate: 78 g (39 g × 2)

Has seeing the calorie count on food packages and posted on menus changed any or many of your food and beverage decisions?

People used to drink juice from 4-ounce juice glasses. Now 10- to 16-ounce glasses and 25-ounce tumblers are typical. No longer is eating on 9-inch plates the norm as it was in the 1960s. Now the average plate size is around 12 inches.

By turning back time, so to speak, and downsizing to the original 9-inch plate, the smaller plate size automatically manages portions and calories. In fact, Brian Wansink,[1] author of *Mindless Eating: Why We Eat More Than We Think*, suggests that swapping a 10-inch plate for a 12-inch plate visually tricks your mind into thinking you're eating more (because the plate looks full), but in fact you eat 22% fewer calories on average. *That could mean, if your typical meal was around 800 calories, simply by downsizing your plate size, you would eat 22% fewer calories and thus could lose around 18 pounds in a year without noticing a big change in your eating.*

Do you remember the partitioned disposable plates that were the norm at picnics in years gone by? They are a little harder to find now, but they do still frequent the shelves of supercenters and can be purchased online. I recall a client I worked with who had type 2 diabetes and was working on weight loss. During his visit, we talked about downsizing his plate to a 9-inch plate, which is the size of the traditional partitioned paper plate. He was intrigued by that idea. So he went

glass or on a large plate, people tend to overserve when using larger glasses and plates. Research confirms that people eat and drink more when they're served larger portions.

[1] Wansink B, Roizen M. *Mindless Dieting: Newsletter #1 in a series* [Internet]. Available from http://mindlesseating.org/pdf/Mindless_Dieting_01.pdf

out and purchased a big package of partitioned 9-inch paper plates. When he returned to see me a couple months later, he had lost about 10 pounds! I asked him what he had been doing differently to result in the weight loss. He said he was eating off the "picnic" paper plates every night (they automatically controlled his portions). He filled the large 1/2 section of the plate with nonstarchy vegetables. One of the 1/4 sections he filled with carbohydrate foods and the other 1/4 section with protein food. He loved the pre-portioned paper plates (and the fact that they saved him from washing dishes as well!). He went on to lose over 30 pounds by using those plates.

Can you downsize your dishes to downsize portions?

> Using larger dishes = Larger portions = More calories = Weight gain

Portion Size Tip #3: Look at the Package Size

In some instances, "individual serving" packages may help control portions, such as choosing 100-calorie packages of almonds (versus eating almonds from a bag and losing track of whether you've eaten 12 or 24 almonds). However, in other instances, a container seen as a single serving may not always be a healthy single-serving portion, such as a pint of sugar-free ice cream. That's where checking out the Nutrition Facts label may help you see that a "single serving" is actually 3 servings.

Become an Illusionist: Smaller Dishes Equal Larger-Appearing Portions

Make visual tricks work for you by using smaller dishes to make portions appear larger, and thus trick your mind into believing you're getting larger portions than you are. Here are some examples of how to trick your mind using plate and glass sizes.

Plate size: 1 cup of black beans and brown rice on an 8-inch plate appears to be a nice size serving. However, 1 cup on a 12-inch plate looks like a little appetizer. The illusion of the "larger" portion on the 8-inch plate will likely leave you feeling more satisfied.

Glass size: With drinking glasses, think slender. A tall, slender 8-ounce glass makes your beverage portion appear larger than it would in a short, wide 8-ounce glass. If you don't fill your glass all the way, studies show you'll tend to pour 30% more into a wide glass than you would into a slender one.

Also, when it comes to package size, studies show that the bigger the package you pour from, the more you will eat—20–30% more for most foods.[2] Think about cereal boxes—pouring from a small box versus pouring from a family-size box. This is one instance where measuring portions can be a big help. You'll find lots of tips a little later in this chapter.

Are a Few Extra Pounds a Concern for You?

Whether you desire to drop a few pounds or proactively prevent weight gain, reducing calories while maintaining a healthful eating pattern is the bottom line. That comes down to managing portion sizes.

Sizing Up Your Portions— Do You Eat More Than You Think?

As famous actor, director, writer, and producer Orson Welles once quipped: "My doctor told me to stop having intimate dinners for four, unless there are three other people." The key message here is to take a look at your portions and size them up. What you may currently think of as a "regular" portion size in fact may not be the "best for you" portion size. *Are your portions too large, too small, or just right?*

---

[2] Wansink B. Can package size accelerate usage volume. *Journal of Marketing* 1996;60(3): 1–14

Practical Methods and Tools to Size Up Portions and Put Them Into Perspective

Many people think they eat less than they actually do. In fact, studies show that people tend to underestimate calories in large meals—the larger the meal, the more the calorie estimation is off. As for carbohydrate control, becoming familiar with serving sizes can help you pinpoint how much you actually eat and whether you are meeting or exceeding your carbohydrate targets. (See more about managing carbohydrate in Chapter 4.)

Going one step further, keep track of the actual portion sizes of what you eat. You may choose to track your food, beverages, and portions through a mobile app, phone Notes, a written log, online, or on the computer—whatever method works for you. And even if you can't track portions every day, any information is better than none. Note any discoveries that you make to share when you meet with your registered dietitian nutritionist (RDN) or diabetes care and education specialist.

To manage portions, you have to first know how much you're eating. The following are three methods to help you size up and manage portion sizes.

Method #1: Measuring Tools

The most accurate way to get familiar with and assess portion sizes is to measure your food or beverage with measuring cups, measuring spoons, or a food scale. Be sure to use liquid measuring cups for liquids (they usually look like a small pitcher) and dry measuring cups for non-liquids—there is a difference. Most people are surprised to see how their actual portion sizes measure up against what they "thought" they were eating. This reminds me of a gentleman I worked with who guessed his cereal bowl held about 1 cup. When he went home, poured cereal in to fill his bowl, and then measured what was in there with dry measuring cups, he found it was actually 2 cups. He discovered he was routinely eating double what he thought.

Let's Practice:

Over the next couple of weeks, measure your food portions as often as possible. The more you actually weigh and measure food, the better you will get at eyeballing portion sizes. You'll soon become familiar with what 1/2 cup of beans looks like on your plate, what 8 ounces of milk looks like in a glass, and what 1 cup of high-fiber breakfast cereal looks like in a bowl.

Top Tips for Measuring Portions

- **Measure your drinking cups and mugs.** Fill your drinking cups with water, and then pour it back into a liquid measuring cup to determine how many ounces your cups hold. You'll then know how much you're drinking when you fill the cup all the way or just part of the way.
- **Measure your bowls**. Fill your bowls with dry cereal and then measure the cereal with a dry measuring cup to identify how much the bowls hold and how much you eat when you fill them up.
- **Measure your plate.** Use a tape measure. Is the plate 9 inches across? Or is it more like 11–12 inches?
- **Use a measuring cup to serve foods** (such as soup, vegetables, casserole, or cereal) rather than using a spoon or ladle. You can then easily quantify the amount you eat and from there determine the carbohydrate count. I gleaned this tip from a client years ago, and it is now a favorite practice among many of my clients.
- **When possible, measure out appropriate individual portions of foods.** For instance, use a measuring cup to put leftover casserole or chili into small plastic containers for reheating so you know exactly how much is in there. Better yet, purchase portion-controlled 1-cup or 2-cup containers. There is no thinking required when you are ready to reheat for lunch or dinner. Measure appropriate portions of nuts, fruit, or other snacks and store them in zip-top plastic bags. That way, you have ready-made grab-and-go snacks.

Let's Practice:

Once a month, do a spot-check to make sure you're still visualizing your portion sizes correctly.

Method #2: Hand Estimations

Although measuring cups and spoons certainly have their place, they aren't always convenient. (Who wants to take measuring cups to a friend's house for dinner? Or to the deli at lunch?) One easy way to get in touch with portions is to use your hand; it's always with you.

Let's Practice:

At a steakhouse-style restaurant. By using your hand to estimate portions, you may find that the sirloin steak you ordered is about 10 ounces (two man-sized palms), that the side of potatoes is about 1 cup (a small adult fist), and the side of dressing for your salad is 3 tablespoons (3 thumbs).

At an Italian restaurant. By using your hand to estimate portions, you learn that the plate arrives with at least 2 cups of cooked spaghetti (two small adult fists' worth). Two cups of pasta is a typical portion size in restaurants. Knowing

---

Using Your Hand to Estimate Portions*

Small adult fist = 1 cup

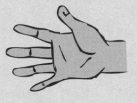

Palm of a woman's hand = 3 ounces
Palm of a man's hand = 5 ounces

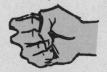

*These are approximations and may vary slightly depending on the size of your hand.

Thumb tip to first joint = 1 tablespoon
Fingertip to first joint = 1 teaspoon
Whole thumb = 1 ounce

Compare your fist size to measuring cups to determine how many cups your fist equates to. Just hold your fist next to the measuring cup, and see how much of your fist will actually fit in the measuring cup. And compare your thumb and thumb tip to measuring spoons to determine how many teaspoons and tablespoons they equate to.

that 1/3 cup cooked spaghetti has 15 grams of carbohydrate (or 1 carbohydrate choice), you realize the 2-cup plate of spaghetti contains 90 grams of carbohydrate (or 6 carbohydrate choices)! No wonder many people notice their blood glucose is above target after eating spaghetti—the portions are often too large.

At a summer barbecue. Using your hand as a guide, you can select a 3-ounce piece of salmon from grilled cedar plank salmon (size of a woman's palm), a cup of grilled veggies (small adult fist), and a teaspoon of margarine (one fingertip to first joint) for your whole-grain roll.

Method #3: Visualize the Right Portion Size

A third method to become familiar with portion sizes is to compare them with everyday objects. Table 7.1 has some of my favorite common comparisons. Once you gain familiarity with standard portion sizes, you can easily compare them to common items and come up with other comparisons that work for you. You can then estimate portions and the associated carbohydrate content.

Let's practice:
Over the next couple weeks as you weigh and measure portions, compare them to common items to begin to build confidence with estimations.

Pre-Portion to Prevent Portion Distortion

Another strategy to manage portion sizes and control the temptation to overeat is to

TABLE 7.1   COMMON COMPARISONS TO FIGURE OUT PORTION SIZES

Portion Size	Common Item
1 slice of whole-grain bread	DVD
3 ounces of meat	Deck of cards
3-ounce fish fillet	Checkbook
2 tablespoons of hummus or peanut butter	Ping pong ball
Medium-size piece of fruit	Tennis ball
1 cup salad greens	Baseball
1/2 cup beans, lentils, or cooked vegetables	1/2 baseball
1/4 cup nuts	Golf ball
1 teaspoon olive oil/ healthy fat	Dice

incorporate pre-portioned foods when possible. You may choose to purchase items pre-portioned, or portion out "right for you" portions into zip-top bags or individual containers at home. I do a combination of both. I buy individual serving cups of yogurt and low-fat cottage cheese, individually wrapped low-fat cheese sticks, and single-serving frozen edamame, for instance. Then pre-portion other foods such as a white chicken chili to have for lunch, or an occasional sweet treat. Pre-portioned foods means no thinking is required when hunger hits.

Here are a few examples of pre-portioned foods you might want to incorporate:

- Naturally pre-portioned apple, clementine, nectarine, orange, pear, or plum
- Instant oatmeal packets
- 100-calorie packs (such as 100-calorie packs of walnuts)
- Individual low-fat Greek or Icelandic yogurt cups
- Laughing Cow or Babybel Light individual light snack cheeses
- Boiled egg
- Foil pack or pop-top can of tuna
- Individual bags of Skinny Pop popcorn

What About Meal Replacements?

A meal replacement is a drink, bar, or shake intended to be used in place of a meal. These portable items usually have controlled amounts of calories, carbohydrate, and other nutrients. Many may be rich in protein or have added fiber. Meal replacements can be helpful if you choose to use them occasionally, particularly when you just don't want to make a decision about what or how much to eat. Meal replacements are portion-controlled, and it's easy to glance at the label and see exactly what nutrients and how much carbohydrate you're getting.

- Individual snack packs of hummus, guacamole, baby carrots, or apple slices
- Healthy frozen meals

Make Swaps to Save Calories Where You Can: Small Calorie Savings Add Up

Granted, trimming portions automatically trims calories. But small switches in the types of foods you eat and beverages you drink can save calories, yet still satisfy your appetite and taste.

If you are trying to cut a few calories to trim a few pounds, saving just 300 calories a day means 2,100 fewer calories to worry about at week's end. And saving 500 calories a day means you're saving 3,500 calories a week. That is definitely a step in the right direction!

In the end, almost any food can fit in your diabetes meal plan in moderation. Moderation is the mantra—the key is how much of a food you eat and how often you eat it.

7 Swaps to Save 100 Calories*

1. Enjoy a small (4-ounce) orange rather than 12 ounces of natural orange juice.
2. Sip on a "tall" (12-ounce), "skinny" mocha coffee drink instead of the regular version.
3. Nestle your lunchtime sandwich between 2 slices of light whole-wheat bread instead of regular bread.
4. Drizzle 3 tablespoons vinaigrette on your salad rather than creamy dressing.

5. Pick a cup of pears canned in juice over those canned in heavy syrup.
6. Savor a spring roll over a fried egg roll.
7. Steam veggies and top with a light drizzle of olive oil rather than sautéing in oil.

---

*Calorie savings are approximate (plus or minus 25 calories).

7 Swaps to Save 200 Calories*

1. Pack flavor in an omelet with 1/4 cup onions and peppers rather than 1/4 cup shredded cheese.
2. Choose a thin whole-wheat or everything bagel in place of a large traditional bagel.
3. Go for 4 ounces of grilled fish instead of fried fish.
4. Dunk a cup of cucumber slices in salsa rather than 18–20 tortilla chips.
5. Crush the chocolate craving with a no-sugar-added frozen fudge pop over 1 cup of chocolate ice cream.
6. Choose 1 cup of mashed cauliflower over buttery mashed potatoes.
7. Munch on two slices of a medium veggie pizza instead of "the meats" pizza.

---

*Calorie savings are approximate (plus or minus 25 calories).

Use a few of the above swaps in 2 days and you'll save 300–500 calories!

Embrace Mindful Eating

Mindful eating means slowing down and being aware and mindful of what and how much you eat, and really tasting and savoring the food.

Pay attention to how you feel. Let hunger and fullness cues help you know when to eat and when you've had enough. Most people find that the first two to three bites bring the most pleasure. After that, what they eat is just "noise," and they don't really enjoy or need any more. The following two strategies can help you to begin to embrace eating more mindfully.

1. Two- to Three-Bite Taste Test

Try the two- to three-bite taste test yourself! A client I worked with for several years loved cheesecake. Before diabetes came into her life, she'd eat an entire giant slice of cheesecake when dining at her favorite restaurant. Once diabetes appeared, she still wanted to try to work in cheesecake on occasion and realized that managing portions was important. She decided to try the two- to three-bite taste test. She reported back that she discovered she really savored the first three bites of her cheesecake, but after that, the pleasure decreased. Based on her discovery, she decided to eat just three bites of cheesecake at the meal, count and incorporate the carbohydrate accordingly, and take the rest home to spread out the pleasure (and carbohydrate) by enjoying two to three bites at several more meals.

2. View It Before You Chew It

It's easy to lose touch with what portion you're eating when eating directly from a bag, box, or carton. I've had a number of clients who loved grapes tell me they could eat a whole 1-pound bag of grapes while watching TV and not even think about it. Each grape has about 1 gram of carbohydrate. Eat 15 grapes, and you've eaten 15 grams of carbohydrate. Eat a pound of grapes . . . well let's just say that's *a lot* of carbohydrate. Another individual I worked with enjoyed eating sunflower seeds out of the shell while reading. She had no idea how many she ate in a sitting. The takeaway is that by portioning what you plan to eat before you eat it, you can see exactly how much you're eating and make adjustments as needed to achieve your carbohydrate target. Leave the package, bag, box, or carton in the kitchen so you're less likely to go back for "just a little bit more." See Table 7.2 for more ideas on how to manage portions that have resonated with my clients over the years.

For additional guidance and support when it comes managing your portions, stay in frequent contact with your RDN. That frequent contact and ongoing education and support are important for consistent and sustained weight loss.

TABLE 7.2　MORE TIPS TO MANAGE PORTIONS

When eating out . . .

- Request a to-go box when placing your meal order, and pack up half of the meal before you begin eating.
- Request a "lunch-size" or "half" portion.
- Order a kid's meal.
- Split an entrée if a dining partner is interested, and order an extra green salad or side of nonstarchy vegetables.
- Opt for soup and a green salad.

When eating in . . .

- Use smaller dishes and more slender glasses so that portions appear larger, but you eat less.
- Serve your plate from the stove. That reduces temptation to eat "just a little bit more."

When eating between meals . . .

- Keep pre-portioned healthy snacks available in portions that fit your carbohydrate and eating pattern (whether you buy them proportioned or do the work yourself).
- For snacks that are not pre-portioned, resist snacking from the bag or package. Rather, place the snack in a bowl or container where you can see what you are actually eating and how much.

Next Steps

Pull out your measuring cups, measuring spoons, and food scale, and begin building your awareness!

1. Measure 1 cup of cold cereal. Pour it into a bowl and notice how it fills the bowl.
2. Weigh a potato that is the size you usually eat.
3. Measure 1/3 cup of cooked brown rice or pasta. Place it on your plate, and compare that with how much pasta or rice you usually eat.
4. Measure 8 ounces of milk in a liquid measuring cup. Pour it into a drinking glass, and note how much it fills the glass.
5. Measure 4 ounces of juice in a liquid measuring cup. Pour it into a glass, and note how much it fills the glass.
6. Weigh a piece of meat, poultry, fish, seafood, or plant-based protein that is the size you usually eat.
7. Measure 1/2 cup of green beans or another nonstarchy vegetable. Place them on your plate, and compare that with how much your typical vegetable portion fills the plate. Do they cover 1/2 the plate?
8. Measure 1 tablespoon of salad dressing. Drizzle it over lettuce, and notice how that compares with the amount of dressing you usually put on salads.
9. Measure out 2 tablespoons of nuts and then 1/4 cup of nuts. Note how those amounts compare to the portion you usually eat.

Food for Thought

- Managing portions is important. Portion sizes are a big concern no matter which eating pattern you embrace, because larger portions mean more calories, more carbohydrate, and thus a greater impact on blood glucose levels and weight.
- Build awareness of portion sizes. Check out available nutrition information. Familiarize yourself with the sizes of your dishes and glasses.
- Use tools of the trade. Use measuring tools, hand estimates, and comparisons of food portions to common household items to determine portion sizes and associated carbohydrate content.
- Use smaller dishes so portions appear larger.
- Use pre-portioned foods when possible.

- View it before you chew it. Put everything you eat in a dish or bowl so you can see exactly how much you're eating and make adjustments as necessary to achieve your carbohydrate targets.
- Make swaps where you can to save calories.
- Embrace mindful eating and remember the two- to three-bite taste test.

PLAN SMART, SHOP SMART, COOK SMART

As you've learned in the previous chapters, what you eat is core to managing diabetes, as well as keeping you healthy and strong. And without a doubt, that takes some thought and time. As I mentioned earlier in this book, evidence shows that following every one of the medical recommendations for diabetes self-care would take at least 143 minutes of your day. That's nearly 2 1/2 hours. And of that time, 57 minutes are related to food—meal planning, grocery shopping, and preparing meals! Knowing what to eat and transforming that knowledge into actually sitting down to enjoy a great-tasting, healthy meal may seem daunting for some. My goal is to help take the stress level down through implementing an abundance of tips I'll share in this chapter to help you plan Diabetes Plate Method meals (whichever eating pattern you're following), shop for those foods, and cook smart. Let's get started with making the most out of those 57 minutes!

Plan Smart

Winston Churchill once said, "Let our advance worrying become advance thinking and planning." *Do you feel anxious sometimes (or all of the time) about when, what, and how much you should be eating?* You can begin to change that anxiety into action by planning meals and snacks in advance. I remember the words of one client with type 2 diabetes with whom I worked. She was an accountant with two young children:

"I've found that if I spend a little time thinking about and preparing food for the week ahead, I make better choices at meals and snack time. If I haven't

thought things through, I find myself heading for the nearest fast-food drive-thru on my way home from work. But if I've got a menu worked out and what I need to prepare a quick and healthy dinner in my kitchen at home, I make much better food choices. Taking a few moments to plan my meals and snacks makes me healthier and often saves me money, too."

This example demonstrates four important benefits of planning meals in advance and reasons to do so:

1. **Healthier food choices.** Taking the time to plan meals in advance can result in meals that align with your eating pattern of choice and follow the Diabetes Plate Method.

2. **Time savings.** A 5- to 10-minute time investment up front to plan meals (and even snacks) will yield greater time savings in the end, because planning enables you to shop for groceries efficiently and avoid extra trips to the store for missing items.

3. **Money savings.** Planning meals ahead means you can create a grocery list and buy only what you need, in the proper package size, so there's less food wasted from extra ingredients that are left over. Also, eating at home, rather than paying for meals out, saves even more money.

4. **Energy savings.** Planning meals in advance not only saves mental energy because you don't have to sweat over what to have for dinner, it saves on

fuel costs by limiting extra trips to pick up forgotten ingredients. I find that cooking is much more enjoyable when I'm prepared.

Planning Meals: Where to Begin?

There's no mystery to designing a plan or "menu" for what you'll eat. All "meal planning" really means is that you decide ahead of time what you'll be eating. You decide how you'll fill the different sections of your Diabetes Plate Method plate. You map out your meals and use them as a guide.

Here are four tried-and-true tips to get started:

1. **Get familiar with the eating pattern you will be embracing.** As a refresher, you can learn more about the different eating patterns to help manage blood glucose in Chapter 3. While this book provides an abundance of basic guidance, I recommend a visit with a registered dietitian nutritionist (RDN), who can review your health and nutrition history, medications, blood glucose patterns, lifestyle, and personal preferences and goals, and then work with you to design an individualized plan. For instance, maybe you've decided to eat more Mediterranean style, but are unsure exactly how many fruits, dairy, and grain foods to aim for each day. An RDN can provide guidance. Once you know the

number of servings of each type of food to try to include each day, you have a basic outline of your meal plan. That outline then translates into your menus (or what you'll eat at each meal and snack), which then becomes your grocery list.

2. **Plan a week in advance if at all possible.** I find it easiest to start by planning dinner. The goal at my house is to plan at least five dinner meals each week, knowing that we may have a meal somewhere else at least one night a week, and the other night we'll repurpose any leftovers (although we do often take leftovers from dinner to work with us for lunch the next day).

3. **Plan with a fresh mind.** I usually plan meals on Saturday mornings when my mind is fresh. Then we grocery shop Saturday or Sunday afternoon. I've found if I try to plan meals after a day at work, I'm tired and not thinking clearly or creatively. *What day and time might work for you to get in the habit of planning, if you're not already doing so?*

4. **Rely on favorites.** Start by thinking about some of your favorite meals and recipes. Note how they fit into your eating patterns. (See Chapter 11 on recipe renewal if you need tips on how to improve the nutritional value of some of those recipes.) These will be the heart of your meal plan. I usually plan meals for the week including two or three that are quick-assembly-type meals (you can learn

more about that later in this chapter) and two or three that may require a little more cooking for the nights we have a little more time to spend in the kitchen. I also frequently incorporate "planned overs." You can learn more about "planned overs" on page 148. There are a variety of recipe and menu planning websites and mobile apps. Some even generate a grocery list for you to simplify things further.

Meal Planning: How To in 5 Steps

Let the Diabetes Plate Method be your guide in meal planning (see Chapter 3 for a refresher). While many start planning a meal based around the protein foods (or entrée), I encourage you to actually start with the nonstarchy vegetables, since they are to fill half the plate. Next, consider protein foods, which should fill about 1/4 of your plate, followed by carbohydrate foods including grains or starchy veggies, then a fruit, and milk/yogurt as your plan allows. If you're not using a meal-planning app, here's how to plan your plate in five steps.

1. Create three columns, either on a piece of paper or electronically. (Many people like to use Excel or a Word document on the computer, so they can easily save the menus and access them to recycle them later on.)

2. In the first column, list five or more nonstarchy vegetables you enjoy.

3. In the second column, list five or more favorite protein foods ("main dishes") you can prepare.

4. In the third column, list carbohydrate foods you'd like to fit in, including grains, starchy vegetables, and then fruit, and milk/yogurt to fit within your carbohydrate goals and eating pattern.

5. Mix and match the items in each column to plan five meals. Once you have the food combinations, you can adjust portion sizes of each to fit the Diabetes Plate Method or your eating pattern.

Expand these meal-planning lists over time with new recipes and other family favorites.

Let's Practice: Carbohydrate-Controlled Mexican-Style Meal

Nonstarchy vegetables (1/2 plate): lettuce, peppers, onions, pico de gallo
Protein (1/4 plate): shredded pork loin
Carbohydrates (1/4 plate): corn tortilla, black beans
Healthy fat: guacamole
Zero-calorie drink: sparkling water with lime

Let's Practice: Mediterranean-Style Meal

Nonstarchy vegetables (1/2 plate): tomato, cucumber, arugula salad with lemon olive oil vinaigrette; steamed broccoli
Protein (1/4 plate): grilled trout
Carbohydrates (1/4 plate): couscous; two small fresh figs
Healthy fat: olive oil on salad
Zero-calorie drink: water

Let's Practice: DASH-Style Meal

Nonstarchy vegetables (1/2 plate): fresh steamed green beans with salt-free seasoning mix; roasted carrots
Protein (1/4 plate): herb grilled chicken breast
Carbohydrates (1/4 plate): wild rice; mixed berries
Healthy fat: olive oil on roasted carrots
Zero-calorie drink: herbal unsweetened iced tea

Let's Practice: Mixed Meal, Spaghetti Dinner

Nonstarchy vegetables (1/2 plate): green salad; marinara for spaghetti
Protein (1/4 plate): ground turkey meatballs
Carbohydrates (1/4 the plate): spaghetti
Healthy fat: Italian or light Caesar dressing
Zero-calorie drink: unsweetened iced tea

"Pick 1–Pick 2" Strategy to Fill Your Plate

If you're looking for additional guidance on more specific portions to fill your Diabetes Plate Method plate, as a place to start, it may be helpful to use what I call the Pick 1–Pick 2 strategy. This plan will give you around 50–65 grams of carbohydrate. Here's how it works:

- **Pick 1–2 grains and/or starchy vegetables/beans = 1 cup total** (approximately 30 grams carbohydrate)
- **Pick 1 protein = 4 ounces** (0 carbohydrate, more if plant-based)
- **Pick 2 or more nonstarchy vegetables = 2 cups total** (approximately 10 grams carbohydrate if raw, 20 grams carbohydrate if cooked)

- **Pick 1 small fruit portion the size of a tennis ball or 1 cup low-fat milk** (approximately 12–15 grams carbohydrate, less if plant-based milk beverage)

Again, this is somewhere to start on your journey to blood glucose management. An RDN can provide guidance on personalizing portions to meet your health and nutrition needs.

3 Strategies to Simplify Meal Planning: Assembly Meals, "Planned Overs," and Backup Meal Plans

When planning meals for the week, I'm a fan of what I call "assembly meals" and "planned overs." Both trim time yet provide a healthy meal that I know my family will enjoy.

Strategy #1: Assembly Meals

There will be those days when you just don't feel like spending a lot of time preparing a meal. That's when I turn to assembly meals, which can take on different forms. Maybe it's a meal prep kit shipped to the front door. Maybe it's a similar meal prep kit purchased at a local market, which is increasingly popular. Or maybe it's a few items you have on hand to pull together a meal in minutes without a lot of preparation.

Here are five assembly meal ideas that you can tweak to suit your needs:

1. **Mediterranean-style stuffed sweet potato.** Microwave a small sweet potato. Split it and top with a foil pack of tuna or reduced-fat feta cheese, sliced red onion, red chiles for a little heat, a squeeze of lime juice, and a dollop of Greek yogurt. Round out the meal with a couple of handfuls of prepared bagged salad greens and a vinaigrette.

2. **Rotisserie chicken meal.** This meal includes purchased rotisserie chicken, steam-in-the-bag fresh or frozen veggies, and bagged kale salad topped with blueberries or strawberries and vinaigrette.

3. **Avocado Caprese salad.** This salad is one of my favorite go-to meals, especially during the summer months. It may sound fancy, but you just layer on your plate sliced tomato, sliced avocado, sliced fresh mozzarella or mozzarella balls, and a few fresh basil leaves or dollop of pesto from a jar. Then drizzle with balsamic vinaigrette (or olive oil and balsamic vinegar) and sprinkle with black pepper. To get in a whole grain, I sometimes layer this over chilled leftover quinoa or add a piece of crusty whole-grain bread.

4. **Plant-based burrito bowl.** Put microwavable quinoa or brown rice (it comes in small, microwavable pouches and individual serving cups) on the bottom of a bowl and top with canned beans (such as black or pinto), salsa (I like to buy and keep fresh salsa or pico de gallo on hand), reduced-fat cheese (dairy or non-dairy), diced avocado, a dollop of reduced-fat sour cream or nonfat

Greek yogurt, and a dash of hot sauce, if you like heat.

5. **Salad with chicken, tuna, or salmon.** Combine bagged salad greens (like kale, spinach, or arugula), cherry or grape tomatoes, purchased fully cooked quinoa (from a cup or pouch), shredded rotisserie chicken or foil-packed tuna or salmon, sliced almonds, and bottled vinaigrette.

Strategy #2: "Planned Overs"

Few people want to eat the same meal day after day, but what I call "planned overs" can become another go-to strategy when planning meals.

Basically, you plan ahead by intentionally making more of an ingredient than you'll eat in one meal and save it to use as part of another meal later in the week. Planned overs can be used for breakfast, lunch, or dinner meals. Use planned overs within 3–4 days or freeze for later use.

Here are five examples of how to create and incorporate planned overs:

1. Roast a turkey breast or cook in a slow cooker. Enjoy as an entrée one day and use the extra meat for turkey pot pie a day or two later.

---

3 Qualities That Make Meals More Appealing

As you launch into planning meals, factor in the following three qualities to make meals appealing.

Color. A colorful plate of food is generally more appealing than a bland plate with everything the same color. We eat with our eyes, so colorful plates are visually more appealing, and a variety of colors generally means a variety of nutrients and better nutrition. *Which looks more appealing?* A meal with chicken, cauliflower, mashed potatoes, and milk (all white), or a meal with chicken, broccoli, sweet potato, and yogurt with blueberries and raspberries (variety of colors)?

Temperature. To add more interest, vary the temperature of your food choices at a meal with some hot foods, some cold foods, and some in-between foods. For instance, tomato basil soup (hot), green salad (cold), and whole-grain crackers (in-between).

Texture. Consider crispy, crunchy, smooth, chunky, and tender foods for your meal menu. Including a variety of different textures generally is more appealing and helps incorporate items from all food groups. For instance, at breakfast, choose nonfat Greek yogurt (creamy) topped with toasted almonds (crispy/crunchy) and fresh peach chunks and blueberries (chunky/tender).

2. Cook extra quinoa, millet, farro, or other whole grain. Enjoy it as a side dish one day, as an addition to Greek-style salad the next, and add to vegetable soup the third day.

3. Roast a chicken or buy a rotisserie chicken. Enjoy it as an entrée one day, as topping for a salad another day for a quick-assembly meal, and in chicken enchiladas the next day.

4. Cook a pork loin in the slow cooker. Enjoy a portion today. Shred some and toss with barbecue sauce to enjoy as pork barbecue at lunch another day.

5. Sauté extra spinach or steam extra broccoli. Enjoy these vegetables at dinner one night and in an egg scramble the next morning.

Strategy #3: Backup Meal Plans

You may find it helpful to have a few backup meals on hand to use when life doesn't go as planned. One night, we'd planned to grill cedar plank salmon, but arrived home from work to a torrential downpour. The salmon stayed in the refrigerator until the next day, and we used a backup meal. Another day we'd planned to have a "planned over" meal with grilled chicken on a green salad. I opened the bag of seemingly fresh salad greens to find many greens were spoiled. Time for another backup meal!

Here are seven backup meal ideas that may inspire you:

1. A foil pack of tuna or salmon, whole-grain crackers, and prepared vegetable or tomato soup

2. Nut butter on whole-grain crackers, baby carrots, and a small piece of fresh fruit or fruit canned in juice

3. Fully cooked shrimp (thaw under cool water and drain well), ready-to-heat quinoa or brown rice, and steam-in-the-bag frozen vegetable

4. A scrambled egg or egg fried in a nonstick skillet; ready-to-heat quinoa or brown rice; frozen vegetables such as spinach, chopped broccoli, onion, or peppers (I keep diced onion and peppers in the freezer for occasions like this); top with salsa or avocado if you have any

5. A panini or oven-toasted sandwich made with whole-grain bread, reduced-fat cheese, fresh vegetables (think tomato, onion, cucumber, zucchini, artichoke hearts, kale, spinach, mushrooms, peppers, etc.), or fresh fruit (such as apples or pears)

6. A healthy frozen meal

7. A planned backup homemade freezer meal (I often stash single servings of leftover bean or lentil soups or chili in the freezer for occasions like this. Or when making a favorite casserole, split a 9 × 13 pan into two square 8 × 8 pans and freeze one to have on hand for a backup meal.)

30 Foods in a Well-Stocked Pantry to Pull Together a Quick Meal

No time to cook? Healthy eating is easier if you keep a variety of basic staple foods on hand to pull together quick and healthy meals and snacks. Then you can add fresh ingredients as needed. The following is a list of 30 foods and ingredients to spark thinking about what you can keep on hand, taking into account your preferences and health goals:

- Applesauce, unsweetened
- Artichoke hearts
- Beans, canned (no-salt-added if possible)
- Cheese, reduced-fat varieties
- Chicken, frozen, fully cooked, diced or sliced
- Coffee
- Cooking spray
- Eggs or liquid egg substitutes
- Fruits, in juice (canned or individual serving cups) or frozen without sugar
- Fruit spreads, 100% fruit or reduced-sugar
- Herbs and spices
- Lentils
- Marinara
- Nuts, including almonds, peanuts, pecans, pistachios, and walnuts
- Nut butter, such as almond butter and peanut butter
- Oil, such as canola or olive
- Pasta, whole-wheat or fiber-enriched
- Red bell peppers, roasted
- Salmon, canned in water or foil-packed
- Salsa
- Shrimp, frozen, fully cooked
- Soups, reduced-sodium and reduced-fat

- Tea
- Tuna, canned in water or foil-packed
- Turkey meatballs, fully cooked, frozen
- Vegetables, a variety of canned or frozen (no-salt-added if possible)
- Vinegars, including balsamic, red wine, and white wine
- Whole grains, fully cooked in microwavable pouches or individual cups (such as brown rice or quinoa)
- Whole-grain bread and crackers
- Yogurt, nonfat or low-fat

Kitchen Tools to Have on Hand

Having the right kitchen tools at your fingertips makes cooking easier and more enjoyable. There is no one ideal list of kitchen tools because the utensils and appliances you need depend on what and how you like to cook. Here are some basics to have on hand to start with:

- Baking dishes, glass and nonstick metal
- Baking sheets, nonstick
- Can opener
- Cutting boards (plastic for meat, wooden for other items)
- Food thermometer
- Grater (box or hand-held)
- Kitchen scale
- Knives (a variety)
- Measuring cups and spoons
- Mixing bowls
- Pastry brush
- Pots (several sizes)

- Roasting pan with rack
- Slotted spoons
- Spatulas
- Strainer

Appliances That Can Be Worth Their Space

Air fryer. If you're someone who enjoys the crisp of fried foods, an air fryer, which "fries" without added fat, may be worth the cabinet space to you.

Blender. Blenders are great for making smoothies, but can be used for a variety of other purposes. For instance, you can use a blender to turn cauliflower into riced cauliflower, frozen bananas into banana soft serve, cooked black beans or pinto beans into puree for bean burgers, and peanuts or almonds into nut butters.

Electric countertop grill. A countertop grill allows for indoor grilling of most any food that could be cooked on a gas or charcoal grill outdoors. One benefit is the fat and juices that cook out can be drained off. Electric grills can also be used to make paninis or other grilled sandwiches.

Food processor. Using a food processor is a fast way to chop, slice, dice, and shred. Other uses include making quick dressings, sauces, and salsas.

Microwave. A standard appliance in most kitchens these days, microwave ovens can be used for thawing, reheating, and cooking countless foods.

Instant pot. An instant pot is a super-speedy pressure cooker that can be used to prepare a variety of foods and meals in minutes.

Most models not only pressure cook, but they also slow cook, steam, and sauté; cook rice and grains; and keep food warm.

Slow cooker. These can be used to prepare a variety of foods with the convenience of putting the food in and then leaving it to cook slowly at a low temperature for several hours. Slow cookers are not only good for soups; due to the low temperature over a long time, they help tenderize less expensive cuts of meat (such as roasts), as well as turkey breasts, chicken, and pork, and even cook oatmeal.

Toaster oven. If you are cooking for one or two, a toaster oven adds the convenience of being able to toast, bake, broil, and warm without heating up the kitchen with the regular oven.

Meal Planning for One

Cooking for one can seem challenging. Here are five tips that have helped many of my clients over the years:

1. **Look for recipes that serve one.** While in years gone by most recipes were designed to feed multiple people, there are now a variety of recipes designed as single servings.

2. **Freeze extra portions.** If buying poultry, fish, or meat, for instance, take out what you'll eat, and freeze the rest in single servings (I use zip-top freezer bags) to pull out for easy use in future meals. Or if making chili, soup, or a casserole, store leftovers in single-serving containers for easy heat-and-eat meals.

3. **Use a toaster oven.** Instead of heating up the big oven, a toaster oven is small, convenient, and quick to heat. Toaster ovens are perfect for roasting a chicken breast, fish, vegetables, baking muffins, and warming leftover portions. Some models are now equipped with an air fryer cooking option in addition to baking and toasting.

4. **Grocery shop at the salad bar.** You can buy exactly the amount you want, and will use, of a variety of vegetables. You can even find things like chickpeas and beets when you'd like some, but don't need a whole can.

5. **Cook once; enjoy twice.** With versatile ingredients like quinoa, cook a little extra to enjoy in a different way (the "planned overs" concept). For instance, an extra cup or two of cooked quinoa can be enjoyed as a savory side dish, a grain salad for lunch, or a breakfast cereal topped with fruit.

Need More Meal Ideas?

Check out *The Complete Month of Meals Collection* published by the American Diabetes Association. It's a unique interactive, three-part, split-page design that lets you create meal plans instantly by mixing and matching breakfast, lunch, and dinner options. Available at www.shopdiabetes.org.

Shop Smart

Diabetes is an expensive condition, which probably goes without saying. Healthcare costs for people with diabetes can be double those for people without diabetes, and most people are looking for any opportunity to save a few dollars. When it comes to food, healthy cooking does not have to cost a lot. This section is designed to share tips to save money and time to get the healthy ingredients you need to prepare healthy meals in your kitchen. Some grocery stores have in-store nutritionists who can provide guidance.

4 Time-Savers of Savvy Shoppers

1. **"Click list" shopping.** Large and small retailers alike offer "click list" shopping, which allows customers to order and purchase groceries online and then pick them up at the store at a designated time, where they're delivered to the car.

2. **Mail-order shopping.** You can buy almost anything online these days, including groceries. In many areas, shoppers can now order groceries online (such as from Amazon) and have them delivered to their doorstep. Or shoppers can use an app to order groceries from select local stores and have them delivered to their home.

3. **Mail-order meal kit delivery.** These meal kits include recipes with the ingredients and are delivered to your door.

4. **CSA memberships.** Community-supported agriculture (CSA) is a way

to buy local food directly from a farmer. You purchase a "share" and become a farm "member." You then receive a box of vegetables or other farm products regularly throughout the growing season. Not only is it convenient, it may help you to eat more vegetables.

6 Money-Saving Tips of Savvy Shoppers

1. **Search for bargains in more than one type of store.**
    - Visit a warehouse club once a month, for instance, to stock up on nonperishable staples in large sizes, and a supercenter for low everyday prices.
    - Check your local food co-op for near-wholesale prices on beans, grains, and other bulk foods.
2. **Minimize the number of minutes spent in the store.**
    - Food marketing research has found that shoppers pay almost $2 for every minute spent inside the grocery store, so getting in and out as efficiently as possible is the goal.
3. **Shop with a list.**
    - The first step to reducing shopping minutes in the store is by shopping with a list to guide you.
    - As you make your list, keep the Diabetes Plate Method in mind. The goal is that about one-half of what's on the list should be nonstarchy vegetables, one-fourth carbohydrate foods (grains, starchy vegetables, beans and lentils, fruits, and dairy), and one-fourth protein foods, with the add-on of healthy fats and zero-calorie drinks or water.
    - Try keeping a running list on your phone's Notes or on the refrigerator door to add to as you realize you need items. Some of my clients have created a "template" of items they typically buy and then fill in items not on the list, or mark off those not needed that week.
    - Organizing your list to match the layout of your grocery store can get you through the store more efficiently and save even more money. Taking this step can prevent time doubling back to pick up forgotten items.
4. **Buy when foods are on sale.**
    - Most grocery stores have predictable sales cycles; for example, perhaps ground beef or certain canned goods are on sale every 6 weeks. Make a note of these sales dates, and then stock up and plan your menus around them.
    - Find out when stores mark down big-ticket items like meat, fish, and poultry. I find that is often on Sunday. If you have adequate freezer space, you can buy and freeze for later use.
    - Buy "in-season" produce. You may find some good buys at the local

farmer's market (while supporting your local farmers). In-season produce is usually less expensive and at peak flavor. Buy only what you can use before it spoils.

5. **Join your store's loyalty program.**
   - Typically signup is free. You then receive electronic coupons and savings when you provide your email address.

6. **Take advantage of specials, coupons, and store brands.**
   - You may find huge deals on specials such as "buy one, get one free."
   - Coupons save money if you use them on items you normally buy. For extra motivation, note the amount you save each week, and use that to treat yourself to a massage, movie, or something else you enjoy.

   - Consumer research shows that store brands or generic versions of products can be of equal or superior quality to name brands and cost 15–30% less. Many of the store brands are made by the same companies that make the big-brand foods.

Cook Smart

What may be holding you back from cooking healthy? Some common barriers I've heard over the years are time, lack of recipes and meal ideas, and low kitchen confidence. You don't have to be a chef to prepare healthy meals. While cooking is a skill, it is a skill that gets better with time and practice. This section includes tips on finding good recipes and making the most of your time in the

---

Cost-Friendly Recipes and Food Plans

The U.S. Department of Agriculture (USDA) has recipes and food plans designed to feed a family of four at home starting at about $150 per week (as of early 2019).

1. Check out the USDA Food Plans Cost of Food page on the USDA website (www.cnpp.usda.gov) for more information and ideas. The USDA also provides lots of recipe ideas on their MyPlate Kitchen page, available at https://www.choosemyplate.gov/myplatekitchen. Many of the recipes can fit within the eating patterns reviewed earlier in this book and have a short ingredient list. Recipes with fewer ingredients are often cheaper and quick to make.
2. Also check out the Healthy Eating on a Budget page at https://www.choosemyplate.gov/eathealthy/budget for many more ideas.
3. See Table 8.1 for more smart shopping ideas.

TABLE 8.1	5 SMART SHOPPING SELECTIONS THAT SAVE MONEY		
Instead of this. . .	Buy this. . .	And save. . .	Takeaway Message
Pre-shredded carrots $0.19/ounce	Whole carrots shredded at home $0.06/ounce	$0.13/ounce	Convenience costs more
Marinated pork tenderloin $4.26/pound	Plain pork tenderloin with spices added at home $3.94/pound	$0.32/pound	Convenience costs more
Brand-name whole-grain toasted oat cereal $0.21/ounce	Store-brand whole-grain toasted oat cereal $0.14/ounce	$0.07/ounce	Brand names cost more
Brand-name olive oil $0.46/ounce	Store-brand olive oil $0.15/ounce	$0.31/ounce	Brand names cost more
100-calorie snack pack of unsalted almonds $0.77/ounce	Bulk-packed unsalted almonds $0.35/ounce	$0.42/ounce	Individual servings cost more

kitchen. I'm a fan of recipes with five ingredients or less. Using recipes with five or less ingredients can make cooking seem more manageable.

Reliable Recipes

One key to being a good cook is having a good recipe. And these days, good recipe resources abound—from YouTube, websites, mobile apps, and cooking shows, to magazines, cookbooks, and more. Many of today's recipes are designed for healthful eating. And for recipes that may not quite meet your preferences and health needs, as you'll learn in Chapter 11 on recipe renewal, small swaps can often renew the recipe.

When checking out recipes, ask yourself the following five questions:

(The goal is to be able to answer "yes" to most or all of the questions.)

1. Does the recipe appeal to your sense of taste?
2. Will the recipe fit into your eating pattern?
3. Is a nutrient analysis of the recipe provided to help you see if/how it fits in your goals?
4. Does the recipe include common familiar ingredients? (Or does it have exotic ingredients that you might only use once or twice?)
5. Does the time required to prep and cook the recipe fit into your schedule?

The American Diabetes Association's website (www.diabetes.org) is a free, rich source of diabetes-friendly recipes complete with nutrition information.

Batch Cooking

Have you heard of batch cooking? Or ever tried it out? Batch cooking simply means making the most of your time in the kitchen by cooking an extra amount of a food for use later (and, yes, batch cooking may intersect with "planned over" meals discussed on page 148).

Five examples of batch cooking:

1. Prepare a double batch of spaghetti sauce. Use half and freeze the remainder to pull out on another day for a dinner that is only a few microwave minutes away.
2. When you have the grill fired up, grill some extra chicken breasts to freeze and thaw later to warm and enjoy on a salad, in a wrap, or as a main dish.
3. While you have the blender out, make a double batch of smoothies, or two different flavors. Portion into small jars with lids, and pop in the freezer to thaw and enjoy later on the run.
4. Make two of a favorite casserole, assembling one in a disposable foil pan. Enjoy one now and freeze the other in the disposable pan to pull out and bake another day. I do this with a favorite chicken and broccoli casserole.
5. Cook a larger roast in the slow cooker. Eat part and then shred and freeze the rest to add to vegetable soup another day.

Batch cooking is a great opportunity to stock the freezer for days when you don't have the time to cook or don't feel like cooking. Some foods are better suited to freezing and reheating than others. Here are a few foods that fare well in the freezer, followed by a few that are best suited *not* to freeze.

Foods to Freeze or Not to Freeze

Freezer-friendly foods:

All of the following foods stand up to the freezer well. Most cooked dishes will keep for 2–3 months in the freezer.

- Baked chicken breasts
- Casseroles
- Chili
- Enchiladas
- Meat loaf
- Pulled pork
- Shredded roast
- Soups
- Spaghetti sauce
- Stuffed peppers
- Tomato sauces

Freezer-unfriendly foods:

- Fruit and vegetables with a high water content, which become watery and limp when frozen (such as cucumber, watermelon, lettuce, or green salads)

- Dishes that have yogurt, sour cream, milk, or light cream as their base; these dairy products will likely separate when frozen
- Cooked pasta and macaroni, which may become rubbery when frozen

Three tried-and-true cooking tips:

In the days of teaching my son some basic cooking, I quickly learned the importance of sharing the following three tips. They may seem basic, but they can help ensure a successful outcome.

1. Read through the recipe at least twice before diving into making it to see if you need to make any swaps, if you have all of the ingredients on hand, and if you understand the steps.
2. Check if you need to do any pre-prep (such as marinating meat) or prepare part of the recipe ahead (such as making a dressing and refrigerating to allow flavors to blend).
3. If it requires an oven or grill, they usually need to be preheated.

Keeping Cooking Safe

The safety we're talking about here is preventing foodborne illness, which can be caused by improper storage or handling of food in the kitchen. The effects of a food-borne illness cannot only rock your intestinal tract and make you miserable, they can have serious effects on your blood glucose. Keep your kitchen safe by properly storing, cooking, and handling your food.

The USDA recommends four easy steps to keep your foods safe:

1. **Clean.** Wash your hands, utensils, and cutting boards often—especially before and after contact with raw meat, poultry, seafood, and eggs. Many people don't realize or think about this. If, for instance, you take raw chicken out of the package to put on the grill, wash your hands immediately or that raw chicken juice on your hands can contaminate everything you touch with salmonella (a common culprit of foodborne illness).
2. **Separate.** Keep raw meat, poultry, and seafood away from foods that won't be cooked. Use separate utensils, dishes, and cutting boards for raw food and cooked foods. Plastic, acrylic, or glass cutting boards are best for meat, since they can be easily washed (as opposed to raw meat juices soaking into wooden cutting boards).
3. **Cook.** Use a food thermometer. The USDA website provides safe cooking temperatures for different foods. You can't tell whether food has been safely cooked just by how it looks. I'll never forget the Thanksgiving my husband smoked a turkey and it looked golden brown, so he declared it done and then took a picture of his prized turkey. But, when he carved into it, it was still raw in the center (although it "looked" cooked from the outside)!
4. **Chill.** Chill leftovers and takeout foods promptly. Discard anything left out

at room temperature for more than 2 hours to prevent foodborne illness. Keep the refrigerator at a safe 40°F or slightly below.

Do you have a food safety question? Check out the USDA website's Food Safety Basics page at https://www.fsis.usda.gov/wps/portal/fsis/topics/food-safety-education/get-answers/food-safety-fact-sheets/safe-food-handling/keep-food-safe-food-safety-basics/ct_index.

Savor the Joy of Eating

While what you eat is core to managing diabetes, as well as keeping you healthy and strong, I encourage you to try to find balance and maintain pleasure in eating. Take time to savor your food and enjoy quality over quantity. I hope as we close out this chapter that you feel better equipped to plan Diabetes Plate Method meals, shop for those foods, and create some delicious meals in your kitchen.

Next Steps

1. Start by planning three menus for the next week. They can be for breakfast, lunch, dinner, or a combination. If you're feeling accomplished with three, then I challenge you to plan a few more.
2. Select one new shopping strategy to try.
3. Find one new recipe that fits your preferences and health goals to try in the next week.
4. Savor the joy of eating!

Food for Thought

- Invest time to plan ahead for meals and snacks to help keep you healthy and strong.
- Save time and money by embracing smart shopping strategies.
- Make cooking manageable by finding some good recipes, keeping a pantry stocked to pull together quick backup meals, and using batch cooking.

HOW TO EAT OUT AND STILL EAT HEALTHY

How often do you find yourself dining out or ordering takeout or delivery? Recent reports show that nearly half of Americans eat out once or twice a week. Without a doubt, eating out is convenient and is often a social experience. Many people ask if managing diabetes means the end to eating out. Of course it doesn't! It is definitely possible to take out or eat out and still manage blood glucose and weight. However, eating out may require a little planning ahead and making a few swaps in what you order. Many restaurants now offer healthy options to try to meet diners' needs, whether they are lower-fat, lower-calorie, lower-carbohydrate, or gluten-free options. This chapter is designed to equip you with a multitude of ideas, strategies, and swaps to keep eating out as healthy as possible.

Planning Ahead Pays Off: 4 Strategies for Eating Out

When did you last eat out? With a little forethought, eating out can be as healthy as it is tasty when you implement a few smart-eating strategies.

Strategy #1: Try to Limit Dining Out Impulsively

Granted, "life happens," and forethought isn't always possible. But when planning ahead is possible, try to select restaurants with a variety of choices, thus increasing your chances of finding foods that work for you.

Strategy #2: Keep 2 or 3 "Go-To" Restaurants at the Front of Your Mind

This is a favorite tip my clients have shared over the years. By having two or three go-to restaurants in mind, which you know have menu options that work for you, when the question arises, *"Where should we meet to eat?"* you are ready with several options to suggest.

Strategy #3: Do Some Restaurant Research

With even a couple of minutes' notice, you can gather information on your dining options and locate healthy options that best fit your calorie, fat, and carbohydrate needs. Otherwise, when defenses are down because you're hungry, "everything looks good."

Here are six tips to keep restaurant research simple:

1. **Check for online menus.** Many restaurants (both dine-in and fast food) post menus and menu items online so that you can identify items that suit your tastes and needs.

2. **Consider calling ahead to see what's on the menu** if going to a new restaurant and you can't locate a menu online.

3. **Look for nutrition information on the restaurant's website (if there is one).** You'll often find nutrition information posted on restaurant websites. Calorie and other nutrition labeling is required for standard menu items in restaurants that are part of a chain with 20 or more locations. Restaurants with fewer than 20 locations may opt in to share nutrition information also. Many fast food restaurant chains also have pamphlets with all the facts and figures you need, which can be especially helpful if you don't go online frequently. Table 9.1 shows you how quickly calories and carbohydrates can add up in a fast-food meal.

TABLE 9.1   FAST-FOOD SURPRISE

Food Item	Calories	Carbohydrate (grams)	Fat (grams)
Crispy chicken sandwich with lettuce, tomato, pickle, and mayonnaise	510	54	20
Baked potato with sour cream and chives	320	62	3
Small chocolate shake	350	58	9
Totals	1,180	174	32

This example shows that *one* typical fast-food meal can contain close to *an entire day's worth* of carbohydrate and fat.

TABLE 9.2	2 SWAPS THAT PAY OFF BIG		
Food Item	Calories	Carbohydrate (grams)	Fat (grams)
Grilled chicken sandwich with lettuce, tomato, pickle, and mayonnaise	370	38	10
Baked potato with sour cream and chives	320	62	3
Small light lemonade	5	1	0
Totals	695	101	13

By making two swaps to the foods listed in Table 9.1, you save 485 calories, 73 grams of carbohydrate, and 19 grams of fat, just by exchanging grilled chicken for the crispy chicken and light lemonade for the milkshake!

4. **Use a free mobile app (there are many) to check out the nutrition information of menu offerings.** There are also many popular restaurants in free online databases such as calorieking.com.

5. **If you prefer a guidebook** to a mobile app, you may want to check out *Eat Out, Eat Well* by Hope Warshaw, MMSc, RD, CDE, or *CalorieKing Calorie, Fat, & Carbohydrate Counter.*

6. **If booking reservations online**, some online restaurant reservation sites will filter dining options based on dietary needs.

Strategy #4: Be Prepared

With the focus on food, as you head out the door, remember to grab any diabetes medications you need to take with the meal and your blood glucose monitor. While there are a variety of special bags and carrying cases designed specifically to keep diabetes supplies together,

I've had clients use zip-top plastic bags, small cosmetics bags, pencil bags, or insulated bags as a simple way to stash and transport everything together.

In Table 9.2, even with the two swaps, the carbohydrate count is still excessive. *How about eating half of the baked potato and taking the other half to go, or sharing it with a dining partner?* That would slash carbohydrate by 31 grams. *Or how about swapping a green side salad with dressing in place of the potato altogether?* That would drop the carbohydrate down much further.

Dash 'N' Dine: Tips to Navigate Fast-Food and Carryout Dining

It's 8:00 a.m., you're late to a meeting, and you didn't have time to prepare breakfast at home. You pull into a fast-food drive-thru to grab a quick breakfast to eat while commuting. After all, you're hungry and know that you need some fuel. A bacon, egg, and cheese biscuit and a medium orange juice are what you order. After consuming 95 grams of carbohydrate, half a day's worth of fat, and just over 650 calories, you're wondering if you should have made a different choice.

How likely is it that you will drive through a fast-food restaurant, grab a carryout meal, visit a food truck, or order food to be delivered to your home sometime in the next week? How about the next month?

When it comes to eating on the run, here are 10 helpful hints to guide you:

Hint #1: Slow Down and Take Timeouts

You may get your food fast, but slow down when it comes to actually eating. Try taking two or three 1-minute "timeouts" to allow your body time to realize you're getting full. Eat for 3–4 minutes and then take a timeout for 1 minute.

Hint #2: Stick with Foods in Their Simplest Forms

An example of sticking to a food in its simplest form is choosing a grilled chicken sandwich rather than processed chicken nuggets.

Hint #3: Go Easy on the Condiments

Just one packet of mayonnaise (about 2 teaspoons) adds 60 calories and 7 grams of fat! Ask if reduced-fat condiments are available. Also, keep in mind that "honey glazed," "honey mustard," and "barbecued" mean extra carbohydrate.

Hint #4: Boycott Breading

When possible, choose foods that are not breaded, or peel off the breading to remove extra carbohydrate (and fat, if it's fried). I've heard many of my patients and clients say they leave off the top or bottom bun on a sandwich to trim carbohydrate and meet their goals.

Hint #5: Eat Like a Kid

"Kids' meals" are a more favorable option for "kids of all ages" as opposed to "value" or combo meal deals. The carbohydrate content and calories in kids' meals are generally much closer to adult mealtime carbohydrate and calorie targets than those in value or combo meal deals. *If you find yourself in a fast-food restaurant and need an easy answer, order the kid-size meal.* See Table 9.3 for more reasons to choose a kids' meal.

TABLE 9.3 IS A MEAL DEAL REALLY A GOOD DEAL?	
"Value Meal"	**"Kids' Meal"**
Quarter-pound burger with cheese	Cheeseburger
Medium fries	Small fries
Unsweetened tea	Unsweetened tea
870 calories	530 calories
83 g carbohydrate	62 g carbohydrate
Swap a "kids' meal" for a "value meal" and save 340 calories and 21 grams of carbohydrate.	

Hint #6: Choose Menu Items Labeled "Small," "Plain," and "Regular"

They are typically the best choices for your health. Alternately, selections labeled "deluxe," "biggie," or "value" mean larger portions and more calories, carbohydrate, fat, and salt.

Hint #7: Select Items on "Dollar" Menus May Be Options

Portion sizes are generally smaller on the "dollar" menu. But if you eat two of those smaller-size sandwiches, for instance, you've defeated your portion-control efforts.

Hint #8: Ask Yourself, "Is a Value Meal Really a Value?"

A "value meal" is not a value and a "meal deal" is not a deal when they contain more food than you need plus empty extra calories and excess carbohydrate and fat. A value meal generally runs around 1,000 calories or higher!

If you feel compelled to order off the value or meal deal menu, try these tips:

- **Share your fries with a dining companion.** Or eat a few and toss the rest, or take them home to reheat and enjoy at another meal.
- **Swap out the fries for a green salad or fruit side option** (now widely available at fast-food establishments). That one switch saves nearly 40–45 grams of carbohydrate and nearly 400 calories.

Hint #9: Keep Salads Healthy

Have you ever ordered a salad at a quick-service restaurant thinking, "It's a salad, so it has to be healthy for me?" Salads seem like a healthy choice, and often are. There are many scrumptious salad alternatives to the traditional burger and fries.

However, loaded salads can bring some surprises:

- **A fast-food taco salad** tips in at about 600–800 calories and 60–70 grams of carbohydrate.
- **A chicken strip salad** (depending on the size and *without* dressing) runs 600–800 calories and 40 or more grams of carbohydrate. The point is, just because "it's a salad" and it has chicken does not always mean it's a healthy choice.

Here are two pointers to help you keep your salads healthy:

1. Stick with salads that are full of lettuce/salad greens and veggies and lean protein (like grilled chicken, salmon, or beans) and drizzled with low-calorie or vinaigrette dressings.

2. Go easy on high-fat and crunchy toppings such as bacon, cheese, croutons, tortilla chips, fried noodles, and regular dressings. They can quickly sabotage your "healthy" salad.

Hint #10: Swap In Thin Crust on Pizza

The thinner the crust, the less carbohydrate. If you're craving a slice of pizza once in a while, here are other pointers to help fit pizza into your meal plan:

- **Choose cauliflower crust,** if that's an option, to cut carbohydrate.
- **Go crustless.** While it may sound impossible, some pizza places offer a crustless pizza where the toppings are instead layered in a small bowl or on a plate.
- **Limit meat toppings** and pile on the veggies instead to reduce fat (see Table 9.4).

Takeaways:

- Swap thin crust for original or deep dish and save big on calories and carbohydrate.
- Swap vegetable toppings for some or all meat toppings, and save big on calories and fat.

Best Bets for Fast Food

I'm not advocating eating fast food frequently, but if you occasionally choose to, it's important to know how to fit it in. Cruising through the drive-thru and wondering what to order? Here are a few of the best bets that can fit in a healthy eating pattern for diabetes.

Fast-Food Breakfast Best Bets

- Oatmeal
- Fruit and yogurt parfait
- Fruit cup
- Veggie Egg White Wake-Up Wrap from Dunkin' Donuts
- Mini Skillet Bowl from Taco Bell
- Spinach, Feta & Cage Free Egg White Wrap from Starbucks
- Reduced-Fat Turkey Bacon & Cage Free Egg White breakfast sandwich from Starbucks
- Protein boxes and bowls from Starbucks

TABLE 9.4   PIZZA COMPARISONS

Thin Crust Versus Original Crust	Calories	Carbohydrate (grams)
Two slices of 12-inch **original-crust** cheese pizza	420	54
Two slices of 12-inch **thin-crust** cheese pizza	310	28
Meat Toppings Versus Vegetable Toppings	Calories	Fat (grams)
Two slices of 12-inch thin-crust **meat** pizza	380	23
Two slices of thin-crust **pepperoni** pizza	320	18
Two slices of 12-inch thin-crust **vegetable** pizza	280	13

- Sous Vide Egg Bites from Starbucks
- Egg White Grill from Chick-fil-A
- Low-fat milk, hot tea, or coffee to drink

Here are a few things to keep in mind when choosing a coffee or tea drink: Black coffee or plain tea are calorie- and carbohydrate-free. However, "doctoring them up" with whole milk/cream, sweeteners, syrups, and whipped topping not only ups the flavor factor, but also ups the calories, carbohydrate, and fat content (see Table 9.5).

Fast-Food and Takeout Lunch-and-Dinner Best Bets

Here are a few of the healthier options for each fast-food and takeout category:

- **Deli sandwich/sub:** Choose a turkey, lean ham, or lean roast beef sub on whole-wheat bread with lots of raw veggies, mustard (spicy or yellow), vinegar, and herb seasoning for flavor. Choose a 6-inch sub over the foot-long version to manage carbohydrate.

---

3 Tips for a Healthier Coffee Drink

1. Opt for nonfat milk or almond milk.
2. If your drink has a flavored syrup, swap in a sugar-free syrup or use fewer pumps.
3. Hold the whipped cream.

TABLE 9.5   COFFEE COMPARISON AT A GLANCE

Type of Coffee Drink (12 ounces; "tall")	Calories	Carbohydrate (grams)	Fat (grams)
Black coffee (or with low-calorie sweetener)	0	0	0
Caffè latte			
With whole milk	180	15	9
With nonfat milk	100	15	0
With soy milk	150	18	4.5
Caramel macchiato			
With whole milk	240	31	9
With nonfat milk	170	31	1.5
With soy milk	190	26	6

Combination Foods and the Diabetes Plate Method

Some foods don't fit exactly on the Diabetes Plate Method. That's OK. Here are two examples of how to fit combination foods in the Diabetes Plate Method

Two slices medium thin-crust vegetable pizza

- *Nonstarchy vegetables (1/2 of the plate)*: veggie toppings (add a green salad to fill the remaining half of the plate and satisfy appetite)
- *Carbohydrates (1/4 of the plate)*: crust
- *Protein (1/4 of the plate)*: cheese (could add ham or chicken for extra protein)

Cheeseburger and side salad (swapped in for fries to decrease the carbohydrate)

- *Nonstarchy vegetables (1/2 of the plate)*: veggie toppings and green salad
- *Carbohydrates (1/4 of the plate)*: bun
- *Protein (1/4 of the plate)*: burger/cheese

- **Chicken:** Try a grilled chicken sandwich with lettuce, tomato, pickle, and light mayo. Choose a multigrain bun if possible.
- **Burger:** Have a junior or kid-size hamburger without cheese or mayonnaise with kid-size small fries, a fruit side, or a green side salad with low-fat dressing. Another option is to choose a veggie burger if available.
- **Pizza:** Go with thin-crust veggie pizza. Opt for ham, Canadian bacon, or chicken if a meat topping is desired.
- **Mexican:** Order soft shells over crispy shells (such as a soft taco or burrito over a chalupa, crunchy taco, or chimichanga). Opt for a veggie and bean or chicken burrito. Choose black beans over refried. Order sour cream and cheese on the side so you can manage the amount you eat. Watch bean, rice, and tortilla chip portions because carbohydrate adds up quickly. As an example:
  - 1/2 cup refried or black beans = 15 grams of carbohydrate
  - 1/2 cup rice = 23 grams of carbohydrate
  - Tortilla chips = about 1 gram of carbohydrate per chip
- **Asian:** Many Asian foods are quite high in sodium, fat, carbohydrate, and calories, so portion control and selection are important.

- Swap out fried entrées with sweet sauces (such as sweet and sour chicken or General Tso's chicken), which are high in fat and carbohydrate. Noodle-based dishes such as chow mein and lo mein are high in carbohydrate, fat, and calories, too.
- Swap in dishes that are rich in vegetables and lean meats (such as fish, shrimp, scallops, chicken, lean beef, and tofu, as long as they are not deep-fried). Vegetable-based entrées can be healthy choices if they are steamed or stir-fried. Shrimp with garlic sauce, moo goo gai pan, and stir-fried mixed vegetables with tofu tend to be among the healthier options.
- Swap in brown rice for white or fried rice; monitor rice portions either way. A 1/2-pint (1-cup) carry-out container of rice has 45 grams of carbohydrate.

Dining Out on Autopilot

Explore and identify a few options at favorite restaurants within your carbohydrate targets to allow occasional dining out on autopilot. Table 9.6 shows an example meal from Wendy's that many of my clients have discovered works for them. It provides 59 grams carbohydrate and 587 calories.

How Does the Meal Affect Blood Glucose?

Check blood glucose 1–2 hours after eating and note the effect. If above your target, consider what you could do differently next time. If in range, great job!

TABLE 9.6   SAMPLE MEAL FROM WENDY'S

Menu Item	Carbohydrate (grams)	Calories
Large chili	23	250
Two packs saltine crackers	9	52
Garden side salad with croutons and ranch dressing	18	250
Apple slices side	9	35
Water or unsweetened tea	0	0

Tip to reduce carbohydrate further: Leave off croutons or crackers.
Tip to swap in healthier fat: Swap out ranch dressing for a vinaigrette.

Other Fast-Food Meals for 45–60 Grams of Carbohydrate

Arby's

Classic roast beef sandwich
Applesauce side
Chopped side salad with light Italian dressing
Water or other zero-calorie beverage

Pizza Hut

Two slices of 12-inch medium Veggie Lovers Thin 'n Crispy pizza
Water or other zero-calorie beverage

Subway

6-inch turkey sub on 9-grain wheat bread, with all vegetable toppings, no cheese,
    and with mustard and vinegar
Unsweetened applesauce or baked chips
Water or other zero-calorie beverage

Have a Seat: 17 In-Restaurant Dining Strategies

When did you last eat out at a restaurant? Getting out of the kitchen to enjoy a meal at a favorite restaurant can be the highlight of the week. *Do you eat the same way at home as in a restaurant? Are the portions the same?* It probably goes without saying that what you choose to order at restaurants can make a big difference. Two common upfront challenges at sit-down restaurants are carbohydrate-rich bread, rolls, or chips that are automatically brought to the table, and larger portions than you may typically eat or want. Here are 17 strategies to keep eating out pleasurable and filled with healthier options.

Strategy #1: Get Ahead of the Game

To avoid waiting for a table, make a reservation or try to avoid times when the restaurant is busiest. If you take diabetes medicines, think about when you'll eat so you can time your medication accordingly.

Strategy #2: Take It Easy on the Bread or Chip Basket

Just one roll, one slice of bread, or 15–20 tortilla chips can add up to 15–20 grams of carbohydrate. Decide whether it's worth "spending" that much carbohydrate before you even start your meal. (If it's a basket of steaming, fresh-baked rolls, you may decide it's worth it.)

Strategy #3: Learn to Understand the Language

Getting familiar with menu terms and cooking basics makes ordering foods easier. Scan the menu for options that are "grilled," "steamed," "broiled," or "baked." Skip "fried" or "breaded" options. Often, foods that are prepared simply (such as steamed, broiled, or grilled items) are lower in fat and calories.

Strategy #4: Do Ask, Do Tell

If you don't know what's in a dish or are not sure of the serving size, ask the server to clarify to help decide if you want to order it or not.

Strategy #5: Practice Meat Mindfulness

To follow the Diabetes Plate Method, order the smallest and leanest cut of meat on the menu, such as a 4-ounce filet rather than a 10-ounce serving of prime rib. Alternately, order a "lunch-size" or half portion if that's an option, split a meat main dish with a dining companion, or take half home for tomorrow's lunch.

Strategy #6: Use Dining Out As an Opportunity to Get a Fish Serving

Over my years in practice, I've heard many clients share that they use dining out as an opportunity to get a fish serving, particularly if they aren't confident in cooking fish or don't want to prepare fish. Their go-to order is grilled, broiled, or blackened fish with a green salad and a non-starchy vegetable side. There is no thinking or carbohydrate counting required, as they know this meal is well within their mealtime carbohydrate target. This thought process aligns with the eating patterns we discussed in Chapter 3.

Strategy #7: Order Creatively

Instead of a dinner entrée, try a salad with a small, light appetizer or a sushi roll (you can order a sushi roll with cooked fish/seafood).

Questions to Ask When Ordering

- Is the soup broth-based or cream-based? (Go with broth-based.)
- How is the meat cooked? Is it prepared with butter, oil, or some other fat? Can the chef go light on that?
- How are the sauces prepared? Can they be served on the side?
- How are the vegetables seasoned? If they are salted, can the salt be left off?
- Can the salad dressing be served on the side?
- What desserts do you offer? Are bite-size or tasting desserts an option?

By deciding in advance whether you'd like to enjoy a dessert or not, you can order the rest of your meal and allocate carbohydrate accordingly to fit the sweet treat in.

At an Italian restaurant, as an alternative to pasta, you may opt for the appetizer meatball (often one or two large meatballs with marinara) and a green salad.

Some appetizer/small-plate favorites to consider:

- Shrimp or crab cocktail
- Bruschetta (a toasted or grilled piece of bread rubbed with garlic and topped with tomatoes, olive oil, and seasonings such as basil or balsamic vinegar)
- Hummus (a chickpea dip made with tahini, olive oil, lemon juice, salt, and garlic) with fresh veggies
- Baba ganoush (a roasted eggplant dip) with fresh veggies
- Lettuce wraps
- Edamame (boiled green soybeans in the pod)
- Meatballs
- California roll (sushi roll containing cucumber, crab, and avocado)
- Seared ahi tuna

Strategy #8: Substitution, Please

If a food doesn't fit into your plan, ask about possible adjustments or substitutions. Instead of carbohydrate-rich rice or the large potato that accompanies your meal, ask for a double order of nonstarchy vegetables, which are lower in carbohydrate. Ask for a low-fat salad dressing rather than the regular variety, or request olive oil and balsamic vinegar to drizzle over your salad. Instead of high-fat sour cream, ask for salsa on your burrito or baked potato.

Special Order!

Making special requests can help maintain the pleasure in eating without guilt or worry about blood glucose swings.

Are you embracing a low-salt/low-sodium way of eating?

- Ask that no salt be added to your food.
- Request condiments on the side so you can manage what and how much extra sodium from them goes on your food.

Are you trying to eat less fat?

- Ask that less or no extra butter be added to your food or that high-fat components of the usual order are on the side or are omitted (so you can manage what you eat).

Are you watching calories and fat?

- Ask that sauces and dressings be served on the side. Drizzle on the amount that fits your eating plan, or dip your fork in the sauce or dressing and then spear your salad or meat.
- Ask about grilled meat, poultry, or fish options (instead of fried).

If you can't get a substitution, then ask if the food be left off your plate to avoid temptation.

Strategy #9: Alcohol: Moderation Is the Mantra

The American Diabetes Association nutrition guidelines advise that people with diabetes limit alcohol. Women who choose to drink alcohol should limit alcohol to one serving or less per day. Men who choose to drink alcohol should limit their consumption to no more than two servings per day. Alcohol has no nutritional value and may disrupt blood glucose, possibly causing it to drop too low (called hypoglycemia). To reduce the risk of hypoglycemia, particularly if you take certain diabetes medications, always drink alcohol with food. Although alcohol itself does not directly raise blood glucose, any carbohydrate in the drink (such as in mixers, beer, and wine) may raise blood glucose. Check out Chapter 12 for more tips on safe alcohol use. Talk with your healthcare team about how to safely incorporate alcohol if you choose to drink.

Strategy #10: Manage Portions

When your food arrives, take note of the portion sizes, how they fill the plate, and the corresponding carbohydrate count. *How do the portions compare to the Diabetes Plate Method and what your plate looks like at home? How does the carbohydrate compare to your carbohydrate goals for the meal?* The portion estimation tips from Chapter 7 may be helpful here. Try to eat the same portions you eat at home.

Strategy #11: Downsize

Large portions are the norm at many restaurants. Take advantage of this by sharing with a dining companion. For example, one person can order an entrée to share, such as grilled fish with vegetables, and the other can order a large green salad. Then, the two of you can share to better manage portions. If you don't have someone to share oversized portions with, or you can't tote leftovers home, then ask for a lunch-size order, half order, or child's meal.

Alcohol Servings

One serving of alcohol has about 100 calories and is equal to:

- 5 ounces of dry wine or champagne
- 3 1/2 ounces of dessert wine
- 12 ounces of beer
- 1 1/2 ounces of distilled liquor (such as gin, rum, vodka, tequila, or whiskey)

Keep in mind that bartenders (and especially home bartenders) frequently serve more than these standard amounts.

Restaurant Best Bets

Here are ideas of what to order to guide you toward eating more nonstarchy vegetables, minimizing added sugars and refined grains, and choosing whole foods over highly processed foods as much as possible. These key factors are common among all of the diabetes-eating patterns.

Appetizers

- Bruschetta
- California roll
- Edamame
- Hummus or baba ganoush with fresh veggies
- Lettuce wraps
- Meatballs
- Seared ahi tuna
- Shrimp or crab cocktail

Salads

- Lettuce or other salad greens and vegetables
- Low-fat dressing on the side (dip fork in dressing before spearing the salad)
- Olive oil and balsamic vinegar with a squeeze of fresh lemon as dressing

Sides

- Roasted, steamed, lightly sautéed, or grilled veggies
- Small portions of potatoes, rice, and noodles/pasta

Entrées

- Grilled, broiled, baked, or roasted fish, poultry, lean beef/lean pork, or seafood
- Sauces on the side
- Vegetable/plant-based dishes that go easy on cheese and/or sauces

Desserts

- Bite-size mini desserts
- Cappuccino
- Fresh fruit
- Sorbet

Strategy #12: To-Go Box, Please

Another way to turn oversized restaurant portions into right-for-you portions is to order a to-go box when you order your meal. Once your meal is served, immediately box up half of it so you won't be tempted to eat "just a little bit more." Now you have tomorrow's lunch or dinner already prepared.

Strategy #13: Add to Your Meal

Look for healthy items you can add to your plate, rather than focusing on what to avoid. Look for nonstarchy vegetables you can add to fill half your plate and for whole-grain sides. Pick dishes that highlight veggies, like a stir-fry, green salad topped with chicken or fish, vegetarian chili, or vegetable-based soup. Order lean meat, poultry, or fish, or a plant-based entrée. Choose foods with healthy fats, such as avocado, nuts, seeds, and olive oil.

Strategy #14: Savor Every Bite

Try to be mindful and pay attention to what you eat to truly enjoy it. Many people find that the first two or three bites are what bring the most taste pleasure. Also, try to stop eating before you actually feel full. It gives your body time to register the feeling of fullness to ward off overeating.

Strategy #15: Practice the Buffet One-Plate Rule

Have you ever overeaten at a buffet (even a seemingly healthy one such as a salad bar)? Or gone back for a second or third plate "to get your money's worth"? Buffets can bring overeating challenges.

Try implementing the "one-plate rule," which works like this: Survey the buffet, ask yourself what items are worth the carbohydrate and calories, grab a plate, and then select the items that you really want (factoring in the carbohydrate count). Put the Diabetes Plate Method into practice, filling 1/2 of your plate with nonstarchy vegetables, 1/4 with carbohydrate foods, and 1/4 with lean or plant-based protein, rather than piling your plate high with foods that you may not really want or need, just because they're there. One plate and you're done. *After all, is a second or third plate really worth it if it will cause you to feel stuffed or experience blood glucose out of range after eating?* Check your blood glucose 1 1/2–2 hours after eating to see how your portions and food choices have affected blood glucose.

Strategy #16: Dessert Dilemma?

With diabetes, dessert isn't necessarily off limits. Sweet treats can be incorporated as part of mealtime carbohydrate. If you would occasionally like a sweet treat, then fit it in by reducing the other carbohydrates in your meal, such as grains, potatoes, bread, or corn. A good approach to "having your cake and eating it, too" is to order one dessert with extra forks and share. Or order bite-size, mini desserts, which are popular on many restaurant menus.

Strategy #17: Rethink Your Drink

Do you drink the same thing at restaurants as at home? Balance out your meal with zero-calorie unsweetened tea, water, sparkling water, or club soda. Add a twist of flavor with a slice of lemon, lime, or orange (which restaurants with a bar usually have readily available).

Surviving Meal Delays

When eating out, among the many variables you may encounter, a big one is that you may end up eating later than usual, or have to wait a while for a table. **Here are a few tips to help keep blood glucose on track if your meal is delayed:**

- **If you know ahead of time** that you will be dining later than usual, you might need a snack at the time you would normally eat the meal. This will help head off hunger and prevent low blood glucose if you take diabetes medicines that may cause low blood glucose.
- **Have treatments for low blood glucose with you** if you take diabetes medicines that can cause low blood glucose. Glucose tablets or packets of gummy fruit snacks are portable and easy to pull out if needed.
- **If mealtime is more than 1 hour late** and your blood glucose is low, treat it as reviewed in Chapter 4 or as directed by your healthcare team. If your

blood glucose is within your target range, but you anticipate it may go low, then eat about 15 grams of carbohydrate (such as three or four glucose tablets or a small roll from the bread basket) to prevent it from dropping too low.

- **If routine mealtime is delayed for more than 1 1/2 hours**, eat or drink a 15-gram carbohydrate snack (such as fruit, fruit juice, milk, or crackers). Consult with your healthcare team on how much carbohydrate to consume for meal delays and when to take your diabetes medications.

See Chapter 10 for additional snacking guidelines and ideas. Check with your healthcare team to determine a game plan for these situations.

Maintain the Pleasure in Eating Out

Eating out is one of life's pleasures. So keep in mind that most any food can fit into your meal plan. You may have to make a few swaps here and there and adjust portion sizes, but by planning ahead and asking for what you need, you can still eat out and manage your blood glucose, too.

Next Steps

1. Practice identifying foods at your favorite takeout or fast-food dining venues that fit the suggested carbohydrate goals for three meals.
2. Think about your favorite restaurant meals, and list two swaps or changes that you can make to these meals so they fit your diabetes eating plan (if there's room for improvement).
3. Check your blood glucose 1 1/2–2 hours after eating out and see if you're in the target range for your blood glucose levels. If not, rethink your portion sizes and carbohydrate estimations. Maybe they were off a bit? If you are in target, then your changes worked. *How can you do more of that?*

Food for Thought

- **Keep two or three "go-to" restaurants at the front of your mind.** Whether dining out is planned or unplanned, you'll have dining options in mind that have menu items that work for you.
- **Do some restaurant research.** Locate healthy options that fit your calorie, fat, and carbohydrate needs so ordering is easier.
- **Make adjustments and swaps** for foods that may not follow your eating pattern and with portion sizes, condiments, and cooking methods to follow the Diabetes Plate Method and keep eating out pleasurable.

SNACK WITH SUCCESS

To Snack or Not to Snack?

Whether in the middle of the afternoon, before bedtime, at the desk, in front of the computer, by the TV, in the car, or at a sporting event, people snack. *Have you ever found yourself munching because you're bored or stressed? Have you caught yourself mindlessly snacking while watching TV?* Snacks have a way of sneaking into life, whether they're planned or not.

Since discovering that you have or are at risk for type 2 diabetes, have you been trying to eat smaller meals with snacks in between in an attempt to regulate your blood glucose? Or have you actually cut out snacking in an attempt to lose a little weight? To snack or not to snack? That is the question!

Snacking: Why, When, and What?

In the past, typical meal plans for type 2 diabetes often called for two or three between-meal snacks each day. It was believed that snacks were necessary to help stabilize blood glucose levels. Now we know that not everyone with diabetes (particularly type 2 diabetes) routinely needs between-meal snacks, especially if three regular meals are part of the day. Extra calories and carbohydrate from unplanned or unnecessary snacks can translate into extra pounds and higher blood glucose. However, snacks may serve several positive purposes for people with diabetes. **This chapter's focus is to bring clarity to three key topics so that you can snack with success:**

- **Why** to snack
- **When** to snack
- **What** to snack on

Why to Snack

Planned snacks (the key word here is "planned") may serve several purposes:

1. To curb appetite and prevent overeating at mealtime
2. To head off hypoglycemia (low blood glucose)
3. To refuel between meals; when meals are delayed; and before, during, and/or after physical activity
4. To boost calorie intake if needed (though most adults with type 2 diabetes are focused on reducing calorie intake to manage weight)

When to Snack

As I alluded to earlier in this chapter, snack times can vary from person to person. While one person may find that a late-morning nibble fuels their pre-lunch exercise class and helps head off hypoglycemia, another may need a small, mid-afternoon munchie to head off pre-supper hunger pangs. And yet another may find that a few bites near bedtime work best. Listen to your body and watch your blood glucose patterns; let them be your guide when it comes to snacking. **Here are three questions to ask yourself when considering a snack:**

1. Are you truly **hungry**? Keep in mind that snacks add extra calories. So if weight loss is one of your goals, plan for those extra snack calories by trimming calories elsewhere in the day.

2. Do you need extra **fuel** for physical activity?
3. Do you need extra **carbohydrate** to keep blood glucose levels in range?

If the answer is "yes" to any of these questions, then it may be time for a snack.

5 Considerations to Help Size Up When You Need a Snack

#1: WEIGHT GOALS

Do you need to lose weight, maintain weight, or gain weight?

- **If you want to lose or maintain weight**, a small, planned, between-meal snack can help curb your appetite and prevent overeating at mealtime. The key is to include the calories and carbohydrate in your daily eating plan to prevent weight gain and/or blood glucose spikes.
- **If you want to gain weight,** those extra calories from snacks can help you achieve your weight-gain goal. Keep in mind, though, that carbohydrate still needs to be counted.

#2: DIABETES MEDICATIONS

If you take any diabetes medications, are you at risk for or do you experience hypoglycemia (low blood glucose) when your medication is at peak action? (If you're not sure, ask your diabetes healthcare team or pharmacist.) **If the answer is "yes,"** a carbohydrate-containing snack can help head off hypoglycemia. And as mentioned above, plan for those extra calories by trimming calories elsewhere in the day. **Here are snacking guidelines to consider based on whether or not you take diabetes medications:**

If you manage your diabetes with insulin or other diabetes medications: Mid-morning or mid-afternoon snacks may be an essential part of your meal plan to help provide energy and prevent hypoglycemia. A snack at bedtime may be called for if your blood glucose levels are below target range (generally <100 mg/dL) or if your blood glucose has a tendency to drop in the middle of the night. It may also be time for a snack if you know you will be eating your next meal later than usual or have unplanned physical activity—that extra bit of fuel will keep your blood glucose from falling too low. Consult your diabetes healthcare team to determine if you should use snacks to prevent hypoglycemia.

If you manage your type 2 diabetes exclusively through healthy eating and physical activity and eat regular meals: Between-meal snacks are not routinely necessary. Your blood glucose is not likely to drop too low, because you are not taking any diabetes medications. However, a snack could be in order for appetite control if your meals are small and hunger hits mid-morning or mid-afternoon, or if you need to fuel up after extra activity.

Consult your diabetes healthcare team for guidance on whether snacks are necessary for you and how to fit them into your meal plan.

#3: BLOOD GLUCOSE PATTERNS

Does your blood glucose log show patterns of low blood glucose at certain times of day? **If the answer is "yes,"** a snack may help head off that hypoglycemia. However, if you take diabetes medicines that can cause hypoglycemia, many healthcare providers prefer to try adjusting medication doses to prevent frequent hypoglycemia rather than encourage additional food intake, particularly if weight control is a concern. Ask your diabetes healthcare team if this applies to you.

#4: ACTIVITY

Do you need extra carbohydrate to fuel physical activity and replenish your energy stores afterward?

- Extra carbohydrate is not usually needed to balance low-to-moderate physical activity of short duration, like a stroll around the block.
- For a higher-intensity and/or longer-duration activity, like a 30-minute jog or a 1-hour cycling class, a carbohydrate snack may in fact be needed before, during, or even after physical activity.

#5: AGE

Do you need extra fuel based on your age and/or appetite?

- Children may need to eat every 3–4 hours because they have small stomachs.

- Teenagers may need extra calories from snacks during the day because they are growing and active.
- Adults may find that a small, planned snack satisfies midday hunger, although some adults can do without snacks. During pregnancy, several small snacks may be preferable and necessary.
- Older adults with small appetites may find they prefer eating small meals with several snacks in between.

What to Snack On

When hunger hits, you may not be sure what to eat. *Should you avoid fruit for snacks? Do you have to eat protein with carbohydrate for a snack? Is a cookie off limits?* The answer to all of these questions is "no!"

When considering potential snack foods, learn as much as you can about their nutrition profile and the amount of carbohydrate in each serving (whether via the Nutrition Facts label, or a mobile app, etc., as reviewed in Chapter 6). Take a look at the fat, sodium, and calories, and try to keep those as low as possible. Compare the standard serving size to the portion size you actually plan to eat, and count the carbohydrate accordingly. *Would you eat one serving? Or two?*

Consider pretzels, for instance: According to the label on the package, one serving of tiny pretzel twists is 1 ounce (17 twists), which contains 23 grams of carbohydrate. If you eat double that serving size (34 twists), then the carbohydrate doubles as well to 46 grams.

Unsure about whether you really need snacks or how to fit them into your eating plan to manage blood glucose? Talk with your diabetes healthcare team about if/when to incorporate snacks to best fuel your body and keep blood glucose levels in range based on your appetite, eating plan, physical activity, diabetes medications, and blood glucose trends. To see how a food and/or beverage affects your blood glucose, check your blood glucose 1 1/2–2 hours later and note the response.

How Much Is Enough?

For most people with type 2 diabetes, a suitable snack typically contains **15–30 grams of carbohydrate.** Check your blood glucose 1 1/2–2 hours after eating a snack to note the impact. (If the snack is used to treat hypoglycemia, recheck your blood glucose 15 minutes after eating to ensure that it has risen above 70 mg/dL. If not, re-treat with another 15 grams of carbohydrate, or as instructed by your diabetes healthcare team.)

Did You Know?

Popcorn is a whole grain. One regular-size bag of microwave popcorn contains 10–12 cups of popped corn. If you eat it all, you crunch down 50–60 grams of carbohydrate. (Kettle corn has even more carbohydrate.) **By switching to "snack-size" or "mini" bags, you can cut carbohydrate in half.**

Snack Myth Busters

Myth: Fruit should not be eaten as a snack.

Fact: One serving of fruit (such as a small orange) is actually a convenient, nutritious, and delicious snack. It contains about 15 grams of carbohydrate—the ideal amount for a small snack.

Myth: If you eat carbohydrate for a snack, you must eat protein with it (such as peanut butter or cheese with crackers) to keep blood glucose levels stable.

Fact: Research shows that in individuals with type 2 diabetes, protein does not increase blood glucose levels or slow the digestion of carbohydrate. Therefore, protein does not have to be eaten with a carbohydrate snack to keep blood glucose stable. Furthermore, adding protein to a carbohydrate snack does not aid in the prevention or treatment of hypoglycemia. Although, a little protein may help promote the feeling of satiety.

Myth: Sweet treats (such as a cookie) are off limits when you have diabetes.

Fact: Current nutrition guidelines for people with diabetes conclude that sugary foods do not have to be avoided, but the carbohydrate in sweets does have to be counted in your meal or snack to prevent out-of-range blood glucose. As reviewed in Chapter 4, sugar is just one type of carbohydrate. Research shows that if the carbohydrate in a sweet treat is counted in the meal or snack and kept within goal levels (or covered with insulin or other glucose-lowering medications), then blood glucose should not be significantly affected.

Select Smart Snacks

When snack time hits, remember the three "S's"—Select Smart Snacks.

Select snacks with these criteria in mind:

- Help maintain blood glucose in range
- Promote health (a great opportunity to work in a fruit or nonstarchy vegetable)
- Tasty
- Satisfying
- Easy to prepare

Selecting smart snacks begins at home. Keeping the pantry and refrigerator stocked with smart snacks means that when hunger hits, you will be prepared. I've compiled a multitude of snack ideas gleaned from clients with diabetes whom I've worked with over the years. I hope you enjoy them, too. Adjust the portion sizes to fit your needs. Snack on!

7 Smart Snacks at Home*

1. Frozen grapes: Remove grapes from stems. Wash and dry grapes well and freeze them on a tray. Then place the grapes in a zip-top bag. They'll remind you of bites of sherbet or sorbet.
2. Frozen 100% fruit juice bars
3. String cheese stick or dill pickle spear wrapped with turkey
4. Air-popped or light microwave popcorn
5. Salsa with cucumber slices for dipping
6. One piece of 100% whole-wheat bread spread with nut butter
7. Smoothie from the freezer

------

*Carbohydrate content varies. Adjust portion sizes to fit your carbohydrate goals.

7 Smart 100-Calorie Snacks*

If calories are a concern and you're trying to keep them in check, try one of these 100-calorie snacks. All of these choices range from 80 to 120 calories:

1. One medium banana
2. 10 large shrimp with 2 tablespoons cocktail sauce
3. 2 tablespoons guacamole and 6 baked tortilla chips
4. Five olives and one mini Babybel light cheese
5. 1/2 cup cottage cheese with 1/4 cup berries (raspberries and blueberries are favorites)
6. 15 almonds
7. 1/2 cup boiled/steamed edamame (green soybeans)

------

*Carbohydrate content varies.

Edamame (Mukimame) Snacks

Buy frozen, steam-in-the-bag, shelled edamame (called *mukimame*), which is widely available in the frozen vegetable section of the supermarket. Microwave according to package directions. Sprinkle lightly with garlic powder or garlic salt and toss to coat. You can also toss with a drizzle of olive oil, flavored oil, or trans fat–free buttery spread. Store in a zip-top bag in the refrigerator. I enjoy it as a snack, a side dish, or tossed in salads.

As an alternative to these 100-calorie snacks, many of the 100-calorie snack packs on the grocery shelves contain 15–20 grams of carbohydrate—just the right amount. Check out the Nutrition Facts label to see which snack packs fit your snack nutrition needs.

7 Smart Snacks to Go*

What do you do when you're on the run and hunger hits? Here are some ideas for portable snacks:

1. Small apple or tangerine
2. Hard-boiled egg
3. Unsalted or lightly salted soy nuts
4. Greek or Icelandic yogurt cup (both are naturally lower in carbohydrate and higher in protein than traditional yogurt)

5. String cheese and a few whole-grain crackers
6. One can of low-sodium tomato or vegetable juice
7. Cherry or grape tomatoes

———————

*Carbohydrate content varies. Adjust portion sizes to fit your carbohydrate goals.

7 DASH-Style Snacks*

1. Pecans
2. Walnuts
3. Broccoli florets
4. Strawberries over low-fat Greek yogurt
5. Oats topped with blueberries
6. Apple slices with peanut butter
7. Grilled pineapple slice

———————

*Carbohydrate content varies. Adjust portion sizes to fit your carbohydrate goals.

7 Mediterranean-Style Snacks*

1. Canned sardines (they work in a fish serving and are portable with the pop-top can)
2. Olives
3. Toothpick skewer of cherry tomato, mozzarella ball, and basil leaf
4. Hummus with baby carrots
5. Baba ganoush with whole-wheat pita bread
6. Roasted chickpeas
7. Avocado slices drizzled with olive oil and balsamic vinegar and a sprinkle of sunflower seeds

———————

*Carbohydrate content varies. Adjust portion sizes to fit your carbohydrate goals.

7 Plant-Based Snacks*

1. Kale chips
2. Red, orange, and yellow pepper strips
3. Almonds
4. Sunflower seeds
5. Pear slices with almond butter
6. Low-fat popcorn
7. Small banana

———————

*Carbohydrate content varies. Adjust portion sizes to fit your carbohydrate goals.

7 Paleo-Style Snacks*

1. Asparagus spears wrapped with prosciutto
2. Toasted pumpkin seeds
3. Grilled peach half
4. Tomato stuffed with egg salad
5. Chia seed pudding (you'll find lots of recipe ideas online)
6. Peanuts
7. Cucumber slices topped with tuna salad

———————

*Carbohydrate content varies. Adjust portion sizes to fit your carbohydrate goals.

7 Very-Low-Carbohydrate (Sometimes Called "Keto") Snacks*

1. Single-serving packets of nut butter
2. Carrot or celery sticks
3. Cucumber boats (split lengthwise, scoop out seeds, and stuff with tuna, turkey, or lean ham)
4. Lower-sodium beef jerky or turkey jerky
5. String cheese
6. Deviled egg
7. Turkey meatballs with marinara

———————

*All contain a minimal amount of carbohydrate. Adjust portions to fit your needs.

7 Smart Snacks for the Workday*

Do you ever get stranded at your desk with no sign of lunch in sight? Stock your desk or workspace with smart snacks that can rescue you. Some people choose to stash only small amounts and restock as needed to reduce any temptation to snack when they're not actually hungry. Also, try to store snacks out of sight to further reduce that temptation.

1. Microwavable containers of vegetable, tomato, or bean soup
2. Unsweetened applesauce cups
3. Fruit cups packed in juice or water
4. Individual packages of nuts (choose heart-healthy almonds, walnuts, pistachios, or peanuts)
5. Foil packs or mini cans of water-packed tuna or salmon
6. Instant oatmeal (plain is lowest in carbohydrate)
7. High-fiber cereal bars

---

*Carbohydrate content varies. Adjust portion sizes to fit your carbohydrate goals.

If you aren't able to fully supply your desk or workspace with snacks from home, don't worry. The following is a list of smart snacks you can pick up at the nearest vending machine:

7 Smart Snacks from the Vending Machine*

1. Small bag of plain pretzels
2. Small bag of peanuts, almonds, or sunflower seeds
3. Small bag of animal crackers
4. Peanut butter or cheese sandwich crackers (whole-wheat varieties if available)
5. Whole-grain cereal bars
6. Wheat crackers (such as Triscuits or Wheat Thins)
7. Cereal mix (such as Chex Mix)

---

*Carbohydrate content varies. Adjust portion sizes to fit your carbohydrate goals.

And here are a few more ideas that you can pick up at the convenience store if that's your best option.

7 Snacks from the Convenience Store*

1. Soft pretzel (if it's huge, share half with a companion or save half for later)
2. Low-fat yogurt
3. Part-skim string cheese
4. Protein bar
5. Can of vegetable or tomato juice
6. Small bag of peanuts, almonds, or sunflower seeds
7. Fresh fruit

---

*Carbohydrate content varies. Adjust portion sizes to fit your carbohydrate goals.

7 Smart "Free" Snacks

If you want to squash hunger without raising blood glucose, try one of the "free" snacks that follow. They're considered "free" because they contain 5 grams or fewer of carbohydrate and fewer than 20 calories per serving.

1. 1/2 cup diced tomato drizzled with 1 teaspoon fat-free Italian dressing

2. 1 cup sugar-free gelatin with 1 teaspoon light whipped topping
3. 1/2 cup baby carrots
4. 1/4 cup blackberries
5. Flavor-infused water, such as the ones described on page 65
6. Mug of low-sodium broth or bouillon
7. Two homemade frozen pops made from a sugar-free fruit drink (such as sugar-free Kool-Aid or Crystal Light)

7 Smart Two-Food-Group Snacks*

Make snack time an opportunity to mix and match. Consider working in two different food groups to ensure the snack provides a variety of nutrients. Snacks are also a great opportunity to work in nonstarchy vegetables, fruit, and dairy servings. Here are some ideas:

1. Apple or pear slices with reduced-fat cheddar or soy cheese
2. Broccoli florets and garlic hummus
3. High-fiber cereal (5 or more grams of fiber per serving) with low-fat milk
4. Peanut butter on a whole-grain toaster waffle
5. Low-fat, no-sugar-added yogurt topped with fruit or as a dip for fresh fruit
6. Whole-grain pita chips and bean dip
7. One date stuffed with almond butter (split date and remove the pit if necessary; stuff with almond butter)

---

*Carbohydrate content varies. Adjust portion sizes to fit your carbohydrate goals.

7 Tips to Crush the Urge to Snack

When you get the urge to munch, it's important to distinguish whether your craving is physiological or psychological. *Are you experiencing actual hunger in your stomach? Are you beginning to feel weak, shaky, or irritable from dropping blood glucose levels?* These are physical cravings that do signal the need for food. Emotions, however, play a big part in snacking, too. Feeling stressed, anxious, frustrated, or lonely can trigger the urge to snack. Even memories of how good certain foods made you feel when you were younger can send you searching for that snack.

Keep in mind, too, that sensory triggers, such as smells and visual cues, can set off cravings. If you leave foods sitting on the counter, then they can trigger the thought that something tasty would be nice. *Have you found yourself wanting a snack while watching a favorite TV program?* Food commercials give you subtle (or not so subtle) reminders to eat.

So, before snagging a snack, think seriously about why you want the snack and whether you really need it. To totally crush the urge to snack (when you don't need the extra calories or carbohydrate), try the following tips that have worked for many clients I've had over the years:

1. Pop a breath mint or breath freshener strip.
2. Use a spray of breath freshener.
3. Chew a piece of sugar-free gum.
4. Rinse your mouth with mint mouthwash or brush your teeth.

5. Suck on ice chips.
6. Take a 5- or 10-minute walk.
7. Drink a large glass of water or another calorie-free beverage.

Top 20 Snacking Strategies

1. **Plan, plan, and plan.** The best snack is one that's incorporated into your eating plan.
2. **Keep an eye on calories.** If you're trying to lose or maintain weight, keep an eye on the calories in the snack portions you eat. For instance, nuts are a healthy snack option. But if you eat 1 cup, that adds nearly 800 calories.
3. **Snack with a reason.** Try to snack only when you're truly hungry or need extra carbohydrate to fuel physical activity or head off hypoglycemia.
4. **Be on guard against stress eating.** When the urge to snack hits you, ask yourself if you are truly hungry (does your stomach feel empty or is it growling?). Eating out of boredom or in response to stress may lead to weight gain and rising blood glucose levels.
5. **Establish a snacking zone.** Eat only at the kitchen table so other locations won't serve as food cues. For instance, if you snack in the recliner in front of the TV, each time you sit there you may find you want to munch on something.
6. **Do away with distractions.** It is too easy to mindlessly overeat while engaged in another activity like working on the computer, playing videogames, watching a movie, or watching TV. When eating, eliminate distractions and focus on your food to help you feel satisfied more quickly and avoid overeating.
7. **If in doubt, keep it out.** If there's a snack food that's too much of a temptation and triggers you to overeat, keep it out of the house. If chips are a weakness, but there aren't any in the house, those fresh fruits or veggies in the fridge may seem more desirable.
8. **Out of sight, out of mind.** Keep snack foods out of sight so you aren't tempted to nibble for no reason.
9. **Make snacks count.** Make snack time an opportunity to work in a fruit, vegetable, milk/milk substitute, or whole-grain serving.
10. **Satisfy sweet cravings with fruit.** When you're craving a sweet and cool treat, try frozen grapes or frozen banana chunks. Eating these foods is an easy way to satisfy your sweet tooth and work in a fruit serving.
11. **Broaden your snacking horizons.** Try something new for snacks. Maybe try soy nuts, a whole-wheat pita bread, or jicama with hummus.
12. **Keep snacking simple and convenient.** Have nutritious, prepared, and ready-to-eat snack options at your fingertips. If fruit and vegetable chunks are conveniently pre-cut, prepared, and in the fridge, you might be more likely to grab them if they're ready to eat.

13. **Love leftovers.** A small serving of last night's entrée or veggie could make an easy, tasty snack.

14. **Watch out for portion distortion.** What is commonly considered a "portion" is often actually more than enough. As reviewed earlier in this chapter, many people think of a bag of microwave popcorn as one "portion." But if you eat the whole bag, that one "portion" actually has 50–60 grams of carbohydrate. Ask yourself whether you really need that many calories or that much carbohydrate.

15. **Keep snacks "snack size."** Smaller, carbohydrate-controlled, snack-size portions can curb hunger without sending blood glucose out of range.

16. **Snack outside the package.** Measure snacks and put an appropriate portion in a bowl or zip-top plastic bag so you know exactly how much you are eating. If you eat directly from a large bag or box, then it's difficult to know exactly how much you've eaten. Did you just eat 10 peanuts or 30? It can be hard to keep track! Studies show that when people eat from bulk-size bags, they eat more.

17. **Single-size can be wise.** Buy snacks in single-serving packages to easily manage portions.

18. **Check out label lingo.** Don't be fooled by labeling claims. Foods marketed as "low-fat" or "fat-free" can still be high in calories and carbohydrate. Check the Nutrition Facts label to find out the whole story.

19. **Make a perfect match.** Match snack calories and carbohydrate to your activity and blood glucose. A marathon runner can consume more calories and carbohydrate than someone who is sedentary.

20. **Enjoy your snack!** Choose snacks that you enjoy. If you don't like raw broccoli, then don't force yourself to eat it.

Next Steps

1. List three snacks you can eat at home that meet your taste and nutrition needs.
2. List three snacks you can eat on the go that meet your taste and nutrition needs.
3. List two strategies you can try to keep snacks and snack portions healthy.

Food for Thought

- Planned snacks can curb your appetite, head off hypoglycemia, refuel your body, and boost calorie intake (for those who need it).
- Not everyone with type 2 diabetes needs snacks. *Do you?* Consult with your healthcare team.
- Depending on your choices, snacks may add extra carbohydrate.
- Know why to snack, when to snack, and what to snack on . . . just for you.

RECESPE RENEWAL

Earlier chapters have provided specific guidance around the balance of nutrients in a healthy eating plan and portioning a plate using the Diabetes Plate Method. Now we're going to turn and focus on recipe renewal. That means learning how to make a few swaps in those favorite recipes that may not align with a diabetes-friendly eating pattern. Many old and beloved family "comfort food" recipes tend to be high in calories, fat, sugar, and salt. In this chapter, you'll glean ideas on how to renew the recipes so that they fit more easily on a Diabetes Plate Method plate.

To recap, here are broad characteristics of a healthy eating pattern/ plan, the goal of which is to help you manage your blood glucose, weight, blood pressure, and lipids:

- Emphasizes a variety of vegetables from all of the subgroups
- Includes fruit, especially whole fruit
- Includes grains, with at least half being whole grains
- Incorporates lower-fat dairy
- Includes a variety of protein foods
- Includes oils instead of solid fats
- Limits solid fats, added sugars, and sodium

Considering those characteristics, here are four questions for you:

1. *What are some comfort foods or indulgent favorite recipes that come to mind that are high in fat, sugar, carbohydrate, or salt and might benefit from renewal?*

189

2. *Do you prepare the food often?* If yes, you might benefit from renewal. If it's a special recipe you only enjoy once or twice year, you may want to leave the recipe as is and just enjoy a smaller portion.
3. *Could you make the recipes healthier by swapping an ingredient or two in each?*
4. *Could you make the recipes healthier by using a different cooking method?*

Keep in mind that the healthy food choices for you are also the basis of healthy eating for everyone around you. So all can benefit from and enjoy renewed recipes!

Ready, Set, Change!

When you set out to revise a recipe, look at each ingredient in the recipe and consider the following:

- **What is that ingredient's function?** *Is it there to add texture? Will the food fall apart if it's not included? Is it there to add color or promote browning? Or is it just a garnish?* If you're not sure, you can learn a little more about the function of different ingredients in recipes as you read through this chapter.
- **Is there one or more swaps you could make to "healthify" the recipe?** You'll see lots of ideas for swaps as you read on.
- **What one swap do you want to start with?** When modifying a recipe, it's important to make only one change at a time so you can note the impact on the recipe's taste, texture, and appearance.

As you make ingredient swaps, take note of both the successful swaps as well as the not-so-great results for future reference. Maybe you learn that when you swap out low-sodium soy sauce for regular soy sauce in a stir-fry, you don't miss any flavor, and that's a successful swap. But maybe when you swap some sugar out of a banana bread recipe, the bread is dry and a little tough. Because that's not the result you were hoping for, you can consider what to do differently next time.

Making Recipes Healthier with Simple Swaps

As mentioned above, make only one swap at a time so you can note the impact on a recipe's taste, texture, and appearance. Let's get started! First up, let's learn how to swap out sugar to reduce carbohydrate in recipes.

How to Swap Out Sugar to Reduce Carbohydrate

Sugar's Function in Foods

Although you may be limiting sugar to help manage your carbohydrate intake, granulated sugar does play a significant role in some recipes (particularly baked goods), and it can't always be fully replaced with another sweetener. Here's what granulated sugar does in cooking:

- **Sugar adds texture, color, and bulk to baked goods.** Substituting other ingredients for sugar in baked goods can cause your cakes, cookies, pies, and candy to turn out very differently than expected.
- **Sugar helps yeast bread rise by providing food for the yeast.** As the yeast grows and multiplies, it uses the sugar and releases carbon dioxide and alcohol, which gives bread its characteristic flavor.
- **Sugar provides the light brown color and crisp feel** to the tops of baked goods, such as muffins and cakes.

Cook's Notes: 3 Strategies to Cut Sugar

1. **How to reduce sugar.** In most cases, you can cut back on the added sugar in your recipe by one-fourth to one-third without a difference in the finished product. If a recipe calls for 1 cup of sugar, for instance, try it with 3/4 cup and note the result. In foods like baked goods where sugar is used to impart texture, refrain from the urge to totally eliminate sugar or totally replace it with a sugar substitute, because your baked goods will not turn out as expected. Some sugar substitutes are not heat-stable, meaning they lose their sweetness when heated, so check the sweetener's label to make sure

it can withstand heat. (See more about the sugar substitutes on page 193 in this chapter.)

2. **Enhance sweetness and flavor with extracts.** You may be familiar with vanilla extract. There is actually a multitude of extracts on the grocery shelves, ranging in flavor from butter to nuts, fruits, liquors, and herbals.

3. **Impart a sweet taste with sweet-flavored spices.** Sweet spices include allspice, anise, caraway, cardamom, cinnamon, chervil, cloves, fennel, nutmeg, and star anise. They add sweet flavor without adding carbohydrate.

While the discussion in this section has focused on sugar thus far, keep in mind that sugar is just one source of carbohydrate. Table 11.1 shows a number of other swaps to consider to reduce carbohydrate in recipes.

What About Sugar Substitutes?

As covered in Chapter 4, "sugar substitutes" refers to high-intensity sweeteners, artificial sweeteners, nonnutritive sweeteners, and other low-calorie sweeteners. The U.S. Food and Drug Administration (FDA) has reviewed a number of sugar substitutes for safety and approved them safe for consumption by the general public, including people with diabetes. The high-intensity sweeteners listed on page 192 are commonly used as sugar substitutes because they are many times sweeter than sugar but contribute few to no calories and carbohydrate when added to foods.

TABLE 11.1   SWAPS TO TRIM SUGAR AND OTHER CARBOHYDRATES

Recipe Ingredient	Healthy Swap
Sugar	1/4 or 1/3 less sugar Sugar baking blend
Sugar added to coffee, tea, or other drinks	Sugar substitute Flavored extract
Bread crumb topping	Ground nuts
Pasta/noodles	Spiralized zucchini or carrots Spaghetti squash Broccoli, cauliflower, spinach, mushrooms, tomatoes, and squash to add flavor and bulk
Cooked rice	Riced cauliflower
Potatoes	Cooked cauliflower (to replace half or more of the potatoes in casseroles or mashed potatoes)
Flour tortillas	Corn tortillas
Pizza crust	Thin crust, flatbread, cauliflower crust, or sweet bell pepper "crust"
Sandwich bread	Low-carbohydrate wrap, large lettuce leaf
Dairy milk	Unsweetened almond or soy milk
Jelly or syrup	Mashed fresh berries or thin apple/pear slices
Fruit canned in heavy syrup	Fruit canned in its own juice or water Fresh fruit

8 Available Sugar Substitutes in the U.S. Include the Following (at Time of Printing)

1. Acesulfame-K
2. Advantame
3. Aspartame
4. Luo han guo (monk fruit extracts)
5. Neotame
6. Saccharin
7. Steviol glycosides (stevia)
8. Sucralose

Table 11.2 provides a brief summary of the available sugar substitutes. In cooking and baking, sugar substitutes may impart a taste difference and impact cooking time as compared to sugar.

TABLE 11.2   COOKING CONSIDERATIONS WHEN USING SUGAR SUBSTITUTES

Sugar Substitute Sweetener	Examples of Brand Names Containing the Sweetener	Cooking Considerations
Acesulfame potassium (Ace-K)	Sweet One Sunette	• 200 times sweeter than table sugar • Stays sweet at high temperatures during baking • Can replace all of the sugar in sauces and beverages, but recipe adjustments may be needed for baked goods
Advantame	(Not sold direct to consumers)	• 20,000 times sweeter than table sugar
Aspartame	Nutrasweet Equal Sugar Twin	• 200 times sweeter than table sugar • Loses sweetness when heated • Won't provide bulk or tenderness in baked goods, so recipe adjustments may be needed
Luo han guo (monk fruit extracts)	Monk Fruit in the Raw PureLo	• 100–250 times sweeter than table sugar • Is heat-stable, so it's suitable for cooking and baking • In baked goods, substitute for up to half of the sugar in the recipe • Works well in beverages, smoothies, sauces, and dressings
Neotame	Newtame	• 7,000–13,000 times sweeter than sugar • Can be used in both hot and cold mixtures as well as for baking
Saccharin	Sweet and Low Sweet'N Low Sweet Twin NectaSweet	• 200–700 times sweeter than sugar • Is heat-stable and can be used in baked goods • Works well in dessert toppings, beverages, and salad dressings

(continued)

TABLE 11.2   COOKING CONSIDERATIONS WHEN USING SUGAR SUBSTITUTES (Continued)

Sugar Substitute Sweetener	Examples of Brand Names Containing the Sweetener	Cooking Considerations
Steviol glycosides (stevia)	Truvia PureVia Enliten	• 200–400 times sweeter than sugar • Stevia-based sweeteners are suitable for baking; however, most can't replace sugar cup-for-cup in recipes. It's best to leave at least 1/4 cup of sugar in the recipe to help with browning and provide texture. • You likely will need to use a lower baking temperature and increase the baking time.
Sucralose	Splenda	• 600 times sweeter than sugar • Retains its sweet taste in a wide variety of temperatures and cooking times • A granulated version measures and pours like sugar and can be used in a variety of ways, including cooking, baking, beverages, sauces, dressings, and frozen desserts.

Sometimes the craving for something sweet strikes. And a chocolate chip cookie would hit the spot. Table 11.3 offers some swaps that can reduce sugar, carbohydrate, and calories and increase fiber and flavor. Make only one swap at a time so you can note the effect.

How to Fix the Fat

Fat's Function in Food

Many recipes won't do well in a totally fat-free world because fat carries out several important functions in food. Here are a few of fat's functions in food:

- Tenderizes
- Adds moisture and shape to baked goods
- Carries and blends flavors
- Adds creaminess to sauces and dips
- Gives a feeling of satiety, making you feel full after you eat
- Carries fat-soluble vitamins and other nutrients

TABLE 11.3 SWAPS TO CHANGE UP CHOCOLATE CHIP COOKIES

Use this. . .	Instead of this. . .	And you get. . .
Dark chocolate chips or mini chocolate chips in 1/2–3/4 the amount	Regular-size chocolate chips	Reduced sugar, carbohydrate, fat, and calories
Uncooked quick oats	Part of the white flour	Increased fiber
Bran cereal (not flakes)	Part of the white flour	Increased fiber
1/4 cup liquid egg substitute	Whole egg	Reduced fat and calories
3/4 cup sugar	1 cup sugar	Reduced sugar, carbohydrate, and calories
3/4 cup sugar + 1/4 cup powdered milk	1 cup sugar	Reduced sugar
Granulated sugar substitute or sugar baking blend	Part of sugar (as per sugar substitute package)	Reduced sugar, carbohydrate, and calories
Double the vanilla or almond extract called for	NA	Increased flavor and sweetness
Add cinnamon	NA	Increased flavor

Cook's Notes: 4 Strategies to Cut Fat in Cooking

1. **Use reduced-fat or nonfat ingredients whenever possible.** For example, swap in low-fat or nonfat Greek or Icelandic yogurt or reduced-fat or fat-free sour cream in place of regular sour cream in dips. Or swap in low-fat milk or nonfat milk for whole milk in pudding.

2. **Skim the fat.** After you make a soup or stew, add ice cubes to congeal the fat on top of the soup for easy skimming. Although the ice will cool the soup, you can quickly rewarm it. Alternately, refrigerate the soup and skim the fat off the top before reheating. Each tablespoon of fat you skim will save more than 130 calories.

3. **Opt out of, or reduce by half, the high-fat, high-calorie extras or toppings in your recipe.** For instance, you may decide to reduce nuts or coconut by half and forgo

altogether a whipped cream topping, a dollop of sour cream, or a sprinkle of cheese.

4. **Use a graham cracker pie crust** in place of a dough pie crust, which is traditionally made with lard or shortening and gets more than half of its calories from fat.

Fat Replacers: At a Glance

You may have heard of fat replacers. As the name implies, they are used to replace part or all of the fat in some foods and thus can reduce fat and calorie intake. The fat replacers currently on the market are considered safe by the U.S. Food and Drug Administration. There are three types of fat replacers used in food products:

- **Carbohydrate-based fat replacers.** Most fat replacers today are made from carbohydrate. Carbohydrate-based fat replacers are made from starchy foods such as grains, corn, cereals, and various fibers, gums, and other starches.
- **Protein-based fat replacers.** These are made by modifying proteins such as egg whites or whey from milk.
- **Fat-based fat replacers.** These are chemically altered fatty acids that provide few or no calories. Some pass through the body virtually unabsorbed.

Takeaways:

- Products made using fat replacers may have less fat and fewer calories, but if you eat a larger portion of a reduced-fat food, you lose any potential calorie savings. Be mindful of portion

sizes and the calorie and carbohydrate content of these products.

- If you are considering using a reduced-fat product, take a close look at its Nutrition Facts label. Products using carbohydrate-based fat replacers can increase the carbohydrate content of the food and can potentially influence your blood glucose.

Your registered dietitian nutritionist (RDN) or diabetes healthcare team can help you decide if including products with fat replacers in your meal plan is the right choice for you.

Remember, fats are the most concentrated source of calories. So cutting fat also cuts calories. Although the end product is likely not exactly the same once fat has been replaced, many fat substitutions produce delicious and moist end products. Table 11.4 shows you the fat facts on three different ranch dressings. Table 11.5 shows us how to swap out a fat for a higher-quality fat (such as those used in the Mediterranean eating pattern).

If you love fried chicken, Table 11.6 offers you a few swaps to give fried chicken a healthy makeover to reduce fat, calories, and sodium, while adding flavor and fiber. Make only one swap at a time so you can note the effect.

Macaroni and cheese is a classic comfort food that's laden with fat and calories. To spark your thinking, Table 11.7 gives you several swaps that can improve the health of the recipe without losing the wonderful cheesy flavor. Make one swap at a time so you can note the effect.

TABLE 11.4   RANCH-STYLE SALAD DRESSING: WHICH WOULD YOU CHOOSE?

	Regular Ranch-Style Salad Dressing	Light Ranch-Style Salad Dressing	Fat-Free Ranch-Style Salad Dressing
Serving size	2 tablespoons	2 tablespoons	2 tablespoons
Carbohydrate (grams)	2	3	11
Fat (grams)	15	7	0
Calories	150	80	50

If reducing fat and calories at the meal is your priority, you may choose the fat-free version. If limiting carbohydrate at the meal is your priority, you may choose the regular version. Or a light version may be a good compromise.

TABLE 11.5   TIPS TO SWAP OUT UNHEALTHY FATS AND LOWER CALORIES

Recipe Ingredient	Healthy Swap
Butter or oil to sauté	Canola oil, olive oil, cooking spray and nonstick pan, or sodium-free broth
Butter or shortening in baking	Replace half with applesauce, mashed bananas, pureed prunes, or pureed pumpkin Add 3 tablespoons ground flaxseed plus 1 tablespoon water in place of each tablespoon of fat or oil
Butter or mayonnaise for spreads	Nonfat or reduced-fat versions Mashed avocado
Whole egg	1/4 cup liquid egg substitute (such as Egg Beaters) Two egg whites
Mayonnaise	Light or low-fat mayonnaise Mashed avocado Hummus

(continued)

TABLE 11.5   TIPS TO SWAP OUT UNHEALTHY FATS AND LOWER CALORIES (Continued)

Recipe Ingredient	Healthy Swap
Heavy cream	Evaporated skim milk Replace half with nonfat plain yogurt
Cream cheese	Reduced-fat or light American Neufchatel Fat-free ricotta cheese Low-fat cottage cheese pureed until smooth
Cream sauce (like alfredo sauce)	Tomato or marinara sauce
Whole milk	2%, 1%, or nonfat milk Fat-free half-and-half
Sour cream	Reduced-fat or nonfat sour cream, Greek yogurt, Icelandic yogurt
Regular cheese	Lower-fat version Use a lesser amount of a stronger-flavored cheese, since a little goes further in flavor (such as swapping sharp cheddar for cheddar)
Bacon	Turkey bacon Canadian bacon Smoked turkey Vegetarian bacon or bacon bits
Ground beef	Extra-lean or lean ground beef Lean ground chicken (without the skin) Lean ground turkey (without the skin) Lentils Mashed black beans
Meat in a casserole	Replace part with vegetables (such as spinach, mushrooms, or eggplant in lasagna), beans, or lentils
Oil in oil-based marinade	Balsamic or other flavored vinegar Citrus juice Nonfat broth

TABLE 11.6   SWAPS TO MAKE FRIED CHICKEN HEALTHIER

Use this. . .	Instead of this. . .	And you get. . .
Skinless chicken	Chicken pieces with skin on	Reduced fat and calories
Nonfat buttermilk to marinate	Whole buttermilk to marinate	Reduced fat and calories
1/4 cup liquid egg substitute or two egg whites	Each whole egg	Reduced fat and calories
Crushed high-fiber cereal (such as Fiber One)	White flour	Increased fiber
Cayenne pepper, paprika, sage	Salt	Reduced salt/sodium and increased flavor
Air frying or baking with cooking spray	Frying	Reduced fat and calories

TABLE 11.7   SWAPS TO MAKE OVER MACARONI AND CHEESE

Use this. . .	Instead of this. . .	And you get. . .
A smaller amount of sharp or extra-sharp cheddar or pepper jack	Cheddar	Reduced fat and calories
Reduced-fat cheese	Full-fat "regular" cheese	Reduced fat and calories
Low-fat cottage cheese or part-skim ricotta cheese	Some of the full-fat cheese	Reduced fat and calories
Light trans fat–free margarine/buttery spread	Butter	Reduced fat and calories
Nonfat milk	Whole milk or cream	Reduced fat and calories
Part-skim ricotta or reduced-fat sour cream	Whole milk, cream, butter	Reduce fat and calories
Whole-wheat or high-fiber pasta	Refined white pasta	Increased fiber
Crushed high-fiber cereal topping	Dry white bread crumb topping	Increased fiber
Pepper, paprika, nutmeg	Salt	Reduced salt/sodium and increased flavor
Broccoli, cauliflower, spinach, mushrooms, tomatoes, and squash	Some of the pasta	Reduced calories, increased fiber and flavor

How to Shake Off Salt

Table salt is the oldest known food additive. Although it occurs naturally to some degree in many foods, most of it sneaks in through packaged and restaurant foods, as well as salt added during cooking or from the salt shaker at the table. Because diabetes can increase the risk for heart disease and kidney disease, you may hear your healthcare team recommending you cut back salt. That's because too much salt can contribute to high blood pressure. Thus, reducing salt intake can be an important strategy for controlling blood pressure to help protect your heart, kidneys, and other organs. The taste for salt is an acquired one, so it can also be unlearned over time. Refer back to Chapter 5 to read more about salt (sodium); there you'll find many more tips and flavor-boosting ideas to trim salt without sacrificing taste.

Salt's Function in Foods

In foods, salt does at least one of the following:

- Helps preserve food
- Adds flavor
- Aids in the rising of yeast breads

Cook's Notes: 5 Strategies to Shake Off Salt

1. **Taste your food before adding salt.** This step may seem logical, but shaking on salt before ever tasting the food can become a habit for some. Removing the salt shaker from the table is a simple way to slash salt intake.

2. **Swap in herbs and spices as a replacement for part or all of the salt in recipes.** Herbs such as basil, bay leaves, dill, parsley, sage, tarragon, and thyme are versatile. Spices such as cayenne, cinnamon, garlic, ginger, black pepper, and lemon pepper are flavorful in a variety of foods. Or switch in one of the many salt-free seasoning blends.

3. **Trim the salt in recipes.** In many recipes, the amount of salt can be cut in half without much change in taste or texture, and in some cases salt can be completely eliminated.

4. **Substitute lower-sodium versions.** A few ideas include using no-salt-added canned vegetables, unsalted stock and broth, reduced-sodium soy sauce, and reduced-sodium seasoning blends.

5. **Cut back on high-sodium foods in your recipes.** You may find you can eliminate, or cut by half, salty recipe ingredients such as ham, pickles, olives, salted nuts, mustard, ketchup, and barbecue sauce.

4 Swaps to Make Over Condiments

Condiments often add a significant amount of sodium. Here are four condiment swaps that lower sodium. These ideas may get you thinking about other swaps you could make.

1. Swap sliced cucumbers for pickles on a sandwich.

Salt Substitutes: At a Glance

What about salt substitutes? Salt substitutes typically come in a shaker and resemble salt. Familiar brands include Morton Salt Substitute and NoSalt. The key difference between salt and salt substitutes is that salt substitutes contain potassium chloride instead of sodium chloride. Potassium chloride tastes somewhat like sodium chloride (salt), although some people note a metallic taste. Be cautious about salt substitutes with potassium chloride. Excess potassium can be harmful if you have kidney problems or certain heart conditions, or if you are taking certain blood pressure medications. Salt substitutes are not a healthy option for everyone. Your RDN or diabetes healthcare team can help you decide if including a salt substitute in your meal plan is the right choice for you. Table 11.8 gives you some tips to reduce salt and swap in flavor in different ways.

TABLE 11.8   TIPS TO SWAP OUT SODIUM/SALT

Recipe Ingredient	Healthy Swap
Salt	Reduce amount by half or eliminate (unless preparing a yeast baked good, which requires salt for leavening)
	Fresh or dried herbs and spices, salt-free seasoning, black pepper, or lemon pepper
	Add aromatic ingredients like onion, green onion, garlic, and ginger
Salt on vegetables	Squeeze of fresh lemon or lime juice
	Splash of flavored vinegar (such as red wine, white wine, balsamic, or rice wine)
Salt in cooking water	Omit the salt when boiling potatoes or cooking pasta, rice, or other grains.
Seasoned salts (such as garlic salt or onion salt)	Salt-free herb and spice seasonings such as garlic powder, onion powder, onion flakes, or celery seed
Soy sauce	Reduced-sodium soy sauce
Broth or stock	Reduced-sodium or unsalted broth or stock
Canned vegetables	No-salt-added canned vegetables and tomato products
	Rinse and drain canned vegetables to remove close to half of the sodium
	Plain frozen vegetables

2. Swap cherry tomatoes for olives at happy hour.
3. Swap whole-grain mustard for yellow mustard (many of the whole-grain or stoneground mustards are lower in sodium per serving).
4. Swap mashed avocado for mayonnaise on a sandwich or burger.

Chili is an ultimate cold-weather comfort food and one-pot meal. It's also an easy slow-cooker meal, and one that freezes well to grab and go on busy days and have in the freezer for backup meals. Table 11.9 gives you a few swaps to keep chili hearty and satisfying, but healthier. Make one swap at a time so you can note the effect.

TABLE 11.9   SWAPS TO MAKE OVER CHILI

Use this. . .	Instead of this. . .	And you get. . .
Chili powder, cumin, and cayenne pepper	Premixed chili seasoning	Reduced sodium, increased flavor
Splash of fresh lime juice or cider vinegar	NA	Brightened flavor
Ground turkey	Part or all of ground beef	Reduced fat and calories
One or more types of beans (pinto, kidney, Great Northern, navy, black beans), rinsed and drained to reduce sodium	Part or all of ground beef	Increased fiber, reduced fat and calories
Whole grains (such as farro, barley, bulgur, or wheat berries)	Part of meat	Increased fiber and flavor, reduced fat and calories
Cubed zucchini, peppers, and carrots in addition to tomatoes	Part or all of meat	Increased fiber and flavor
No-salt-added canned tomatoes	Regular canned tomatoes	Reduced sodium
Fresh toppings such as chopped avocado, cilantro, and diced red onion	Shredded cheese	Reduced fat and calories
Nonfat Greek yogurt or sour cream for topping	Sour cream	Reduced fat and calories

Green bean casserole has been a favorite found on many tables, especially during the holiday season, for over 50 years. This dish is traditionally made with canned green beans, canned cream soup, milk, sour cream, and canned fried onions. Table 11.10 shows a few swaps to reduce sodium, saturated fat, and calories. Make one swap at a time and note the effect.

How to Fit in More Fiber

Fiber is loaded with health benefits (see Chapter 5 for more information on fiber and tips to increase fiber in your eating plan). Because most Americans get less than half the daily recommended amount of fiber, fitting more fiber into recipes is a good strategy for better health.

TABLE 11.10 SWAPS TO MAKE OVER OLD-FASHIONED GREEN BEAN CASSEROLE		
Use this. . .	**Instead of this. . .**	**And you get. . .**
Steam-in-the-bag green beans or no-salt-added canned green beans	Regular canned green beans	Reduced sodium
Reduced-sodium, reduced-fat cream of mushroom soup (such as Campbell's Healthy Request)	Regular cream of mushroom soup	Reduced saturated fat and sodium
Nonfat milk or unsweetened almond milk	Whole milk	Reduced fat and calories
Light sour cream	Regular sour cream	Reduced fat and calories
Chow mein noodles	Canned fried onions	Reduced fat and calories
1/2 the amount of fried onions, crushed (covers casserole to impart flavor with less)	Regular amount of canned fried onions	Reduced fat and calories
Fresh onions lightly sautéed or roasted/carmelized with a splash of olive oil	Regular canned fried onions	Reduced fat and calories
Toasted sliced almonds	1/2 or all of regular canned fried onions	Reduced saturated fat

Cook's Notes: 3 Strategies to Fit in More Fiber

1. **Look for opportunities to fit in more vegetables (especially nonstarchy vegetables).** An example of fitting in more vegetables could be simply increasing the amount the recipe calls for (such as extra tomatoes or beans in chili, maybe in place of part of the beef). You could also top thin-crust pizza with peppers, onions, mushrooms, tomatoes, and hot peppers in place of meat toppings. Or you could fit in vegetables in unique ways (such as adding grated carrot to meatloaf, grated zucchini in a casserole, chopped broccoli or spinach to scrambled eggs, or kale to a smoothie).

2. **Bring on the beans.** Both cooked dried beans and canned beans are an excellent source of fiber. Drain and rinse canned beans to remove around 40% of the sodium.

3. **Experiment with a variety of whole grains.** Barley, buckwheat, bulgur, millet, quinoa, sorghum, and whole rye are all whole grains that can lend fiber and a different flavor profile to recipes—in place of white rice, for instance. To save time, cook extra and freeze in portions to use later as a quick side dish.

With even one intentional swap, you can fit more fiber into a variety of recipes from breakfast to lunch or supper. Table 11.11 shows

TABLE 11.11   SWAPS TO FIT IN MORE FIBER

Recipe Ingredient	Healthy Swap
All-purpose flour	Whole-wheat flour replacing 1/4 to 1/2 of all-purpose flour
White rice	Barley, brown rice, farro, or quinoa
White pasta	Whole-wheat or fiber-enriched pasta
Bread crumbs (as a binder)	Rolled oats, instant barley, or almond meal
White bread or breadcrumbs	Whole-wheat or whole-grain bread or breadcrumbs
Ground beef	Replace half with cooked beans such as pinto beans, black beans, kidney beans, or Great Northern beans (if canned, drain and rinse to remove nearly half the sodium)
Fresh fruit, peeled	Fresh fruit with edible peels left on (such as apples, pears, peaches, and plums)

you a few swaps to get you on the way to filling up with more fiber.

Switching out a few ingredients in a muffin recipe or "quick bread," such as banana bread, can increase fiber and reduce sugar, calories, and fat. Make one swap at a time and note the effect (Table 11.12).

Take a look at a simple recipe for making French toast; think about some easy changes you can make to reduce the fat, sugar, and salt while increasing the fiber and flavor. Table 11.13 gives a list of common French toast ingredients and swaps you can make to

the recipe. Make one swap at a time and note the effect.

How to Fortify Flavor

No matter how healthy the recipe, good taste and flavor are the most important ingredients. Consumer research shows that taste is actually the main reason Americans favor one food over another. With that said, it stands to reason that if you're reducing some ingredients in a recipe to cut back on fat, sugar, and salt, you may need to fortify flavor in other ways. Good-for-you foods should taste good, too.

TABLE 11.12	SWAPS TO MAKE OVER MUFFINS OR BANANA BREAD	
Use this. . .	**Instead of this. . .**	**And you get. . .**
Whole-wheat flour	All-purpose flour (swap for up to 1/2)	Increased fiber
1/4–1/2 cup mashed banana	1/4–1/2 cup oil	Increased flavor, reduced fat and calories
1/4–1/2 cup unsweetened applesauce	1/4–1/2 the oil	Reduced fat and calories
1/4 cup liquid egg substitute	One whole egg	Reduced fat and calories
Two egg whites	One whole egg	Reduced fat and calories
Double the vanilla extract	NA	Increased flavor
Almond extract (start with 1/4–1/2 teaspoon)	NA	Increased flavor
1/2 cup finely grated carrot	NA	Increased fiber, flavor, and moisture
1/4–1/3 less sugar + sugar baking blend	Full amount of sugar	Reduced sugar, carbohydrate, and calories

TABLE 11.13   SWAPS TO TURN AROUND FRENCH TOAST

Use this. . .	Instead of this. . .	And you get. . .
100% whole-wheat bread	White bread	Increased fiber
Low-fat or nonfat milk	Whole milk	Reduced fat and calories
1/4 cup liquid egg substitute OR Two egg whites	One whole egg	Reduced fat and calories
1/2 teaspoon salt	1 teaspoon salt	Reduced salt/sodium
1 teaspoon extract (vanilla, almond, maple, raspberry, strawberry)	Sugar	Reduced sugar, carbohydrate, and calories; increased flavor
Cinnamon	NA	Increased flavor
Fresh berries or unsweetened frozen berries, thawed	Regular syrup	Increased fiber, decreased sugar
Sugar-free syrup	Regular syrup	Reduced sugar and calories

Cook's Notes: 5 Tips to Enrich and Enhance Flavor

1. **Start with the freshest ingredients.** While fresh fruits and vegetables are ideal, frozen versions are generally frozen immediately after picking, so they retain flavor better than the canned, processed versions. Also, they're lower in sodium. You may consider a patio or backyard garden, frequenting the local farmer's market, or joining community-supported agriculture (CSA) with a local farm to access the freshest and locally grown produce.

2. **Experiment with herbs.** For easy access, you may choose to have a windowsill herb garden or try out the popular aerogardening. Aerogardens are foolproof, dirt-free, indoor gardens where you can grow a variety of herbs, vegetables, and other plants. Either way, you can have fresh herbs to snip. Here are three tips on how to incorporate herbs:
    ○ Keep in mind that dry herbs have stronger flavor than fresh herbs. So if using dry herbs, swap 1 teaspoon of a dried herb in place of 1 tablespoon of the fresh variety.

- ○ For chilled foods, such as salad dressings and dips, add herbs several hours before serving to allow time for their flavors to blend.
- ○ For hot dishes, such as soups or sauces, add herbs toward the end of the cooking time, so the flavor doesn't cook away.

3. **Pep up flavor with peppers.** Try fresh green, red, yellow, and orange peppers of all types, from sweet to heat. Use fresh or dried peppers. Or add a dash of hot pepper sauce.

4. **Add tang with grated lemon, lime, or orange peel or juice.** The acidic ingredients help elevate and balance flavor with minimal calories.

5. **Add a burst of flavor with an intensely flavored condiment.** Fresh fruit or vegetable salsa, horseradish, and wasabi are three ways to add flavor without lots of sodium, fat, or calories.

A Few More Swaps for Mediterranean, Plant-Based, and Reduced-Carbohydrate Eating Patterns

Tables 11.14 through 11.16 show several swaps to make to match certain eating plans.

Make Recipes Healthier by How You Cook Them

Changing the way you cook a food can significantly reduce fat and calories, making

TABLE 11.14 8 SWAPS TO MAKE A RECIPE MORE MEDITERRANEAN-STYLE

Recipe Ingredient	Healthy Swap
Beef	Chicken or fish
Butter	Olive oil
Vegetable oil	Olive oil
Butter or melted cheese on vegetables	Tomato sauce with herbs or marinara
Sandwich roll or bun	Whole-wheat pita
Jelly or jam	Fresh berries
Salt	Basil, mint, ginger, or paprika
Mayonnaise as a spread	Mashed avocado

TABLE 11.15 6 SWAPS TO MAKE A RECIPE MORE PLANT-BASED

Recipe Ingredient	Healthy Swap
Butter	Blended or mashed avocado
Cow's milk	Almond or soy milk
Dairy yogurt	Soy yogurt
Ground beef	Beans and legumes
Sour cream– or mayonnaise-based dip	Hummus
Beef or chicken broth	Vegetable broth

TABLE 11.16   5 SWAPS TO REDUCE CARBOHYDRATE IN RECIPES

Recipe Ingredient	Healthy Swap
Pasta	Zucchini noodles or spaghetti squash
White rice	Riced cauliflower
Bread crumbs	Almond meal
Banana in a smoothie	1/2 an avocado
Tortilla, sandwich bun, or bread	Lettuce leaf wrap

TABLE 11.17   WORST, BETTER, AND BEST COOKING METHODS

Worst	Better	Best
Pan-fried	Lightly stir-fry (with small amounts of oil)	Air-fry
Deep-fried	Lightly sauté (with small amounts of oil)	Bake Broil Grill Microwave Nonstick skillet with cooking spray Poach Roast Steam

it a healthier option. For instance, switching from pan-fried pork loin chops to grilled pork loin chops takes you from one of the unhealthiest cooking methods to the healthiest. In Table 11.17, you see other better and best cooking methods in comparison to the worst-for-your-health cooking methods.

Swap Out the Basting Liquid

If the recipe directions call for basting the meat or vegetables in oil or drippings, use a small amount of nonfat vegetable broth or dry wine.

Next Steps

1. List five favorite recipes that you could renew by making a few ingredient swaps.
2. Pick one to work on first. Then decide what you can swap to reduce fat, sugar, carbohydrate, or salt and/or increase fiber and flavor.
3. Make just one change at a time and note the effect so you can decide if it worked for you or if you want to go back and try something different.

Food for Thought

- Favorite recipes can be renewed, or "made over," to decrease the fat, sugar, carbohydrate, and salt content and increase the fiber and flavor.
- Consider each ingredient in the recipe and its function. Can the ingredient be swapped or changed and still yield a flavorful recipe?
- Think of the kitchen as somewhat of a cooking "lab" where you can experiment at making modifications.
- Make one swap at a time so you can note the effect and determine whether the change works for you.

SPECIAL OCCASION STRATEGIES

Special occasions are an important part of life—be it holiday gatherings, parties, family celebrations, potlucks, a toast to an accomplishment, or a trip. Each brings unique eating opportunities and challenges. *How has diabetes affected the way you celebrate at these different events?*

This chapter is designed to equip you with a multitude of practical strategies and tips to successfully navigate a variety of situations, including:

- Holidays, parties, and social gatherings
- Family celebrations and potlucks
- Alcohol consumption
- Travel

Holidays, Parties, and Social Gatherings

Since diabetes (or prediabetes) showed up, have you ever felt like skipping out on holiday feasts, church socials, birthday parties, or other special events because of potential eating challenges? Granted, these types of situations can be tough. Not only are there many different foods you are unsure about, but well-meaning family and friends may sometimes say upsetting things or police what you eat.

There are things you can do to help plan for these events. With a few strategies in place, you will find with time that you can make it through most any social situation. After each event, reflect on what went well and how you can repeat that at future gatherings. Also think about what didn't go as planned and what changes you can make at future gatherings to keep your blood glucose in range.

**Social Gathering Strategy #1:
Take Something Healthy to Share**

If you are concerned that the food at the gathering will be laden with carbohydrate, fat, and calories, then consider offering to bring a

healthier dish to share that suits your preferences and needs. That way you'll know there's at least one item you can enjoy without worry. And chances are, your host will welcome an addition to the party spread.

A Colorful Vegetable Platter to Share

One colorful healthy option to take to the next social gathering is a vegetable platter. Taking this platter can help ensure that you have a low-carbohydrate option and meet the goal of covering half your plate with nonstarchy vegetables. You can purchase a pre-made vegetable platter. However, you can also quickly put one together including both familiar vegetables as well as a variety of others for a taste twist. See Table 12.1 for some vegetable ideas. For convenience, you may choose to purchase some of the vegetables already prepped and cut up.

Rather than compartmentalizing each type of vegetable, jam everything possible onto a colorful plate or platter, using a bit of care to make sure that colors are spaced out and that all the vegetables are showing their best side. Scatter two or three small bowls of flavored hummus, guacamole, or olive tapenade throughout for dunking the vegetables.

TABLE 12.1   VEGETABLE OPTIONS TO INCLUDE ON YOUR PARTY PLATTER

For a Taste Twist	Familiar Standbys
Asparagus of different colors (lightly steamed and chilled)	Broccoli florets
Baby corn	Cauliflower florets
Broccoli rabe or broccolini (lightly steamed)	Celery sticks
Cherry or grape tomatoes (of different colors if available)	Baby carrots
Edamame (soybeans in the pod)	Cucumber sticks or slices
Jicama sticks	
Red, green, yellow, and orange bell pepper strips	
Sugar snap peas	
Zucchini or summer squash strips	

Social Gathering Strategy #2: Consider Eating a Small Snack to Curb Your Appetite Before the Event

Some people find it helpful to eat a small snack before heading out to the festivities. If you've had a snack, you can focus on fun and visiting, rather than being sidetracked by your appetite, concerns about food options that work for you, and potential worry about blood glucose dropping out of range.

---

3 Small Pre-Party Snack Ideas

1. Small handful or walnuts, peanuts, pistachios, or almonds
2. Single-serve cup of Greek or Icelandic yogurt
3. Stick of string cheese

Social Gathering Strategy #3: Take a Cruise (Along the Party Spread, That Is!)

Before filling your plate with a little bit of everything, cruise the buffet or party spread to see what's available, and then decide which foods you really want, and what portion of each best fits your carbohydrate goals. Ask yourself, *"Is it worth the carbohydrate or calories?"* If the answer is "no," then it may be best to pass it by. If the answer is "yes," then decide what portion

fits your carbohydrate budget before adding it to your plate.

Social Gathering Strategy #4: Fill Half of Your Plate with Vegetables

Aim to fill at least half of your plate with nonstarchy veggies. (If you bring the vegetable platter mentioned earlier, then you've got this covered.) Raw vegetables will keep you munching and fill you up with minimal carbohydrate and calories, leaving room in your carbohydrate budget to sample some special foods.

Social Gathering Strategy #5: Plan Ahead to Incorporate High-Carbohydrate Foods

Have you ever tried to trick yourself into believing that "just a little bit" of a carbohydrate-rich food won't affect your blood glucose? The reality is that that strategy often doesn't work out so well. However, by planning for and incorporating the carbohydrate from the treat or special food, rather than simply adding it onto your meal, you can still enjoy it and manage blood glucose.

Social Gathering Strategy #6: Go For Protein If You Can

When you're cruising the spread, take note of protein options. Maybe there's cheese, nuts, chicken salad, or sliced turkey or beef that can curb hunger with little carbohydrate or effect on blood glucose.

Craving a Sweet Treat?

When the craving for a sweet treat strikes, you can satisfy your sweet tooth with the following sweet treats for about 15 grams of carbohydrate each. Of course I'm not advocating that you eat candy; however, the practical me wants to share the best way to fit candy in, if you do opt for a sweet treat.

- 21 M&M's
- 8 pieces of candy corn
- 3 Hershey's Miniatures candy bars
- 6 jelly beans
- 1 fun-size Milky Way bar
- 3 red-and-white peppermint or cinnamon hard candy discs
- 1 fun-size Twix
- 10 Whoppers (one small pouch)

Social Gathering Strategy #7: Stick with Tiny Tastings of Foods That Are Not Familiar

Many of my clients over the years have shared success with keeping their blood glucose in range by sticking with tiny tastings of foods they may not be familiar with or sure of exactly what's in them. When taking small portions of these foods, they can still enjoy the experience without too much worry of sending their blood glucose out of range. This strategy is also great when traveling and sampling foods of different cultures.

Social Gathering Strategy #8: Plan for Alcohol If You Choose to Drink

Decide your limit on alcohol before any special occasion. Consider starting with a non-alcoholic beverage (especially if you're thirsty) and then slowly savor your alcoholic beverage of choice. If you choose to have more than one alcoholic drink, make the drink in between nonalcoholic. Choose maybe club soda or sparkling water. That way, you'll give your body time to process the alcohol you've already consumed. The big thing to know is that alcohol may cause your blood glucose to drop too low, especially if you take diabetes medications that have hypoglycemia as a side effect (check with your pharmacist if you're not sure). Extra physical activity and dancing may intensify the effect. More information on incorporating alcohol safely (if you choose to drink it) follows on page 216, under Alcohol and Diabetes: How Do They Mix?

Social Gathering Strategy #9: Include a Walk or Other Type of Physical Activity During the Day

Given that physical activity lowers blood glucose, intentionally fitting in a walk or other physical activity the day of a special event can help keep blood glucose stay in range if food choices end in a bit of a splurge.

Are the Calories Worth It?

Are the party foods worth the amount of activity necessary to burn off the extra calories?

A 150-pound woman would have to:

- Walk about 30 minutes at 3 miles per hour to burn off one 12-ounce light beer.
- Dance energetically for about 40 minutes to burn off one slice of apple pie.
- Cycle for about 10 minutes to burn off a 1-ounce cube of cheese.

When Heading out the Door to the Festivities, Remember to Take:

- Any diabetes medicines you'll need.
- Your blood glucose meter and supplies.
- A quick-acting carbohydrate source, such as glucose tablets (especially if you take glucose-lowering medicines).

Some find peace of mind in stashing a carbohydrate snack or two in their pocket or bag as a backup, just in case eating is delayed or there aren't options they prefer.

What About Family Celebrations and Potlucks?

Think back to the last family event you joined. Was it a holiday gathering, a picnic, or a family reunion? Many family gatherings, mine included, are potlucks, or everybody brings something to

4 Snacks to Pack and Go

1. Protein bar
2. Nuts
3. Chewy granola bar
4. Four-pack of cheese crackers or peanut butter crackers

contribute to the meal. *What are some challenges you've had at potlucks? Did you eat more than usual?* In addition to the tips shared above, here are four strategies to make eating at family celebrations and potlucks a little bit easier.

Celebration and Potluck Strategy #1: Use a Smaller Plate to Manage Portions

While the original disposable paper plates were about 9 inches across, these days, platter plates abound. If you find yourself facing a platter, see if there are smaller plates available (maybe for salads or desserts), and use that smaller plate. It will help you manage portions.

Celebration and Potluck Strategy #2: Skip Second Helpings

This really goes without saying. Focus on filling your plate the first time around with foods that are enjoyable yet manage carbohydrate, and skip a second trip.

Do your best to follow the Diabetes Plate Method. Potlucks and family celebrations often are heavy on rich casseroles. Look for nonstarchy vegetables and veggie salads to fill half your plate, and then meats/proteins. Hold starchy carbohydrate-rich foods to one-fourth of the plate. I once had a client who greatly enjoyed indulging in fried chicken at church potlucks. We talked about the Diabetes Plate Method and keeping the chicken to filling one-fourth of the plate. He then inquired how high he could pile the chicken in that section of the plate! If you too are asking that question, the best bet is to stack food no higher than a deck of cards.

Celebration and Potluck Strategy #3: Enjoy Tastings of Special Foods

Try to choose small portions of special foods, and save things you eat every day for every day.

Celebration and Potluck Strategy #4: Take a Healthier Version of a Favorite

If old-fashioned green bean casserole is a family favorite, for instance, consider one or two swaps you could incorporate to make this dish healthier. Check out Chapter 11 on recipe renewal for lots of ideas. Maybe you swap in no-salt-added canned green beans for the regular version and reduced-sodium, reduced-fat cream of mushroom soup (such as Campbell's Healthy Request) for the regular variety.

Alcohol and Diabetes: How Do They Mix?

Whether it's a beer with friends after work, a glass of wine at a dinner party, or a champagne toast on New Year's Eve, alcoholic beverages are frequently part of today's social life. So you may be wondering how alcohol and diabetes mix. Ultimately alcohol intake is an individual choice, taking into account any potential medication interactions. If you like to enjoy an occasional alcoholic beverage, the good news is that you most likely can continue to do so (unless some of your medications or other health conditions prevent it). Moderation is the key. As noted earlier in this chapter, the *American Diabetes Association recommends no more than one alcoholic drink per day for women and no more than two per day for men.* This consumption is moderate and sensible and generally has minimal short- or long-term negative effects on blood glucose in adults with type 2 diabetes. In fact, some data show improved blood glucose and insulin sensitivity with moderate intake. (However, evidence does *not* suggest to start consuming alcohol if you don't already.) That said, more than three drinks a day for men (or 21 drinks a week) and more than two drinks a day for women (or 14 drinks a week) on a consistent basis may contribute to elevated blood glucose.

What Counts As One Drink?

One alcoholic drink has about 100 calories and is equal to:

- 12 ounces of beer
- 5 ounces of dry red or white wine
- 5 ounces of champagne
- 1 1/2 ounces of distilled spirits
- 3 1/2 ounces of dessert wine

3 Considerations if you choose to sip an occasional alcoholic beverage:

1. Calories
2. Carbohydrate
3. Potential increased risk for hypoglycemia

Calories Count

Alcohol has no real nutritional value, but you do need to factor in the calories, especially if you are trying to lose weight. Check out the calories in the three common mixed drinks below. These are 4-ounce portions, so you may need to double or triple the calories and carbohydrate amounts given, depending on the size of the beverage you are served.

- **4-ounce margarita**—185 calories and 16 grams of carbohydrate
- **4-ounce cosmopolitan**—213 calories and 13 grams of carbohydrate
- **4-ounce daiquiri**—224 calories and 9 grams of carbohydrate

Consider as well that alcohol consumption reduces inhibitions and self-control, which may lead to munching down more calories and carbohydrate than planned.

Carbohydrate Can Be a Concern

Distilled Spirits and Mixed Drinks

When it comes to carbohydrate, straight distilled spirits (including gin, rum, tequila, vodka, and whiskey) do not have any carbohydrate and thus do not directly affect blood glucose levels. However, the carbohydrate in mixed drinks *can* raise your blood glucose. For instance, a 4-ounce mojito made with rum contains 16 grams of carbohydrate. You saw other examples previously.

Wine and Champagne

Dry wines and champagne have minimal carbohydrate, although sweet dessert wines are a different story. For sweet dessert wines, you'll have to count the equivalent of 1 carbohydrate choice (15 grams of carbohydrate) for a 5-ounce glass.

Beer

Light beers (<4.5% alcohol by volume) and low-carbohydrate beers are lower in carbohydrate than regular or dark beers. Per 12-ounce serving, light beers are equivalent to 1/2 carbohydrate choice (about 7.5 grams of carbohydrate), whereas regular beer is 1 carbohydrate choice (15 grams of carbohydrate) and dark beers are 1–1 1/2 carbohydrate choices.

Risk for Low Blood Glucose with Alcohol

As mentioned earlier in this chapter, moderate alcohol consumption generally has a minimal effect on blood glucose in people with type 2 diabetes (with the exception of carbohydrate-rich beverages). However, it's important to be aware of the potential increased risk for hypoglycemia (including during the night or fasting the next morning) when consuming alcohol, especially if taking diabetes medications for which hypoglycemia is a side effect or if using insulin. Why? Very simply put, one of your liver's jobs is to put out glucose to help maintain your blood glucose levels, but when you drink alcohol, the liver switches priority to processing the alcohol, and thus glucose output is decreased. As a result, blood glucose levels may drop—sometimes too low.

Consuming alcohol with food and more frequent blood glucose monitoring can minimize the risk of hypoglycemia while sleeping.

Talk with your pharmacist if you are unsure if this may be a risk for you if you take diabetes medications.

An Ounce of Prevention

If you choose to drink alcohol, here are a few tips to help minimize any problems:

- **Have a plan.** Discuss with your healthcare team how to safely fit in alcohol based on your diabetes management plan.
- **If low, then "no go."** Do not drink alcohol if you have low blood glucose because the alcohol may drop it further.
- **Manage portions.** Limit alcohol to no more than one drink a day if you're a woman and two drinks a day or fewer if you're a man.
- **Wear a diabetes ID of some type.** Wearing an ID will help prevent any confusion and keep you safe if you

---

Symptoms and Treatment of Hypoglycemia (Blood Glucose Below 70 mg/dL)

Symptoms of hypoglycemia include feeling shaky, weak, sweaty, clammy, confused, nervous or anxious, irritable, dizzy or lightheaded, or hungry or having a fast heartbeat. If experiencing these symptoms, try to check your blood glucose if possible. If not, it's best to assume your blood glucose is low (below 70 mg/dL). **Treat with 15 grams of carbohydrate** (such as three to four glucose tablets, an individual tube of glucose gel, 4 ounces of juice or regular soda, or 1 tablespoon or sugar, honey, or corn syrup). Wait 15 minutes and recheck. If your blood glucose level is still below 70 mg/dL, re-treat with another 15 grams of carbohydrate.

should experience hypoglycemia, since symptoms of low blood glucose can mimic signs of intoxication.

Alcohol Strategy #1

To manage carbohydrate and calories from alcoholic beverages, choose light or low-carbohydrate beer, dry white or red wine, dry champagne, or "skinny" mixed drinks (meaning drinks with low-calorie/low-carbohydrate mixers). Carbohydrate-free mixers include club soda, diet sodas, and diet tonic water.

Alcohol Strategy #2

To reduce the risk of low blood glucose, particularly if you take insulin or other glucose-lowering medications, never drink alcohol on an empty stomach.

Alcohol Strategy #3

To find out how alcohol affects you, keep a close watch on your blood glucose levels by checking more frequently than usual, checking before you go to bed, and possibly even setting an alarm to wake you up to check during the night. Remember the potential increased risk for hypoglycemia (including during the night or fasting the next morning) when consuming alcohol, especially if taking diabetes medications with hypoglycemia as a side effect, or if using insulin.

- If your blood glucose approaches 70 mg/dL or below and it's not mealtime, eat a 15- to 30-gram carbohydrate snack.
- If you don't typically eat a bedtime snack, but you take diabetes medications and your blood glucose is <100 mg/dL at bedtime, then eat a

---

Swaps to Reduce Carbohydrate in Alcoholic Beverages

Swap in these lower-carbohydrate options	Swap out these higher-carbohydrate options
Light or low-carbohydrate beer	Regular or dark beer
Dry white or red wine	Sweet wine or wine coolers
Dry champagne	Sweet champagne
Distilled liquors, straight (such as bourbon, gin, rum, scotch, or vodka) or "skinny" cocktails	Mixed drinks with sweet, sugar-containing mixers or liqueurs (such as daiquiris, margaritas, mojitos, and sweet martinis)

15- to 30-gram carbohydrate snack. Keep a snack that does not require refrigeration by your bed so you don't have to get up if you need it. Easy snack ideas for this purpose include juice boxes, peanut butter crackers, or a granola bar.

Most important, consult with your diabetes healthcare team about how to personalize these recommendations to suit you.

Alcohol Alternatives

Looking for a lower-alcohol alternative? Try:

- A wine spritzer. Mix two parts wine with one part club soda.
- Choose beer with a lower alcohol content.
- Dilute mixed drinks with club soda, seltzer, or extra ice.

Looking for nonalcoholic alternatives? Try:

- Club soda, sparkling water, or water with a twist of lemon, lime, or orange
- Diet tonic water with a twist of lime
- Diet soda with a twist of lemon, lime, or orange
- Nonalcoholic beer
- "Virgin" cocktails

Travel with Success

Whether your itinerary includes a short road trip, cruising to an exotic port, or flying to the far corners of the Earth, traveling with diabetes and maintaining healthy eating practices can be a pretty smooth ride with a little planning ahead. The following five tips can help navigate travel-related eating challenges to manage diabetes successfully.

Travel Tip #1: Do Some Investigative Work

If you are traveling on a plane or train, check when you make the reservations to see if a meal, snack, or beverage will be offered. Before your travels begin, see what food establishments and markets will be close at hand both during your travels and once you reach your destination. Err on the side of caution and don't count on foods and beverages always being readily available; have a stash with you. (See the list of "20 Travel-Friendly Foods," which follows, for some ideas that have worked for clients I've worked with over the years.) And because traveling and eating out typically go hand in hand, put the tips discussed in Chapter 9 to the test during your trip.

Travel Tip #2: Enjoy Local Specialties

When trying out local cuisine, one of the most important tips is portion control. Many people have shared success with keeping their blood glucose in range by sticking with tiny tastings of unfamiliar foods. Make your best estimate as to the portion that meets your carbohydrate needs, and then check your blood glucose 1 1/2–2 hours after eating to see how the food affects you. If your blood glucose is out of range, take a walk or do some type of physical activity to help lower it. If you take rapid-acting insulin based on blood glucose levels, then make appropriate adjustments as advised by your diabetes healthcare team. Talk in advance with your diabetes healthcare team about how to handle this type of scenario before you depart for your trip. Learn from the situation, so you'll know what to expect if you choose to eat the food again.

Travel Tip #3: Ask for a Refrigerator and/or Microwave in Your Room

Many hotels can provide a small refrigerator or microwave upon request. That way you can keep a few snacks or beverages chilled, or prepare instant oats or a cup of soup, for instance.

Travel Tip #4: Ask Restaurants for What You Need

Restaurants can usually accommodate many of your needs. For instance, you might want to request an egg or oats rather than pastries for breakfast.

Travel Tip #5: Take a Test Drive

Test your travel plan by taking a short weekend road trip (before tackling a 2-week trek across the globe, for example) to master the eating and diabetes challenges that accompany travel.

20 Travel-Friendly Foods

Travel with portable, ready-to-eat snacks in case of meal delays or food unavailability. The following are examples, depending on your travel scenario:

1. Individual portions of nut butter (such as almond butter or peanut butter)
2. Nut butter sandwich (natural almond butter or peanut butter on whole-grain bread)
3. Whole-grain crackers or a mini 100% whole-wheat bagel with nut butter
4. Vacuum-packed tuna or salmon packets and whole-grain crackers
5. Reduced-sodium turkey jerky
6. Individual-portioned packs or zip-top bags of almonds, pistachios, peanuts, soy nuts, or roasted pumpkin seeds
7. Small packs or zip-top bags filled with high-fiber cereal
8. Homemade or store-bought trail mix in zip-top bags
9. Fresh fruit (apple, small banana, clementines, or pear, or zip-top bags of grapes, cherries, or berries)
10. Single-serving containers of unsweetened applesauce or fruit packed in juice
11. Small boxes of raisins or craisins
12. Raw vegetables in zip-top bags or individual-portioned packs (baby carrots, celery sticks, grape tomatoes) with single-serving cups of hummus or guacamole
13. Low-fat popcorn in a zip-top bag

14. Cereal bars or granola bars (choose those with 5 grams of fiber or more per serving)
15. Protein bars (choose those that fit within your carbohydrate goals with minimal to no added sugar)
16. Single-serving beverages (bottled water, low-fat milk boxes, 100% juice boxes, or canned tomato juice or vegetable juice)
17. Single-serving low-fat Greek or Icelandic yogurt cups
18. Cheese and crackers (whole-grain crackers with low-fat string cheese)
19. Individually wrapped reduced-fat cheeses
20. Boiled eggs

To prevent food spoilage, use a small cooler bag with freezer packs for transporting perishable foods. A favorite trick of mine is to fill empty water bottles 3/4 full of water and freeze for disposable "ice packs." Perishable foods should not be kept at room temperature for longer than 2 hours total.

10 Tips to Travel Well with Diabetes

Tip #1: Wear a diabetes ID. Wearing an ID (bracelet, necklace, wristband, etc.) that says you have diabetes and notes if you take insulin can speak for you when you cannot.

Tip #2: Over-pack your medicines and diabetes supplies. You never know when you'll run into a travel delay, so the rule of thumb is to pack *double* the amount of medicine and supplies you think you'll need. Gone for 5 days? Pack 10 days' worth.

Tip #3: Ease through airports. Before air travel, you can always check with the Transportation Security Administration (TSA) for the latest travel updates and to learn about current screening policies (visit www.tsa.gov). Tell the TSA agents that you have diabetes. A note from your doctor explaining your diabetes supplies, medicines, devices, and any allergies may come in handy.

Tip #4: Keep your medicines and supplies close by. Pack them in your carry-on bag to keep them temperature-controlled, prevent damage, and avoid losing them in transit. Insulin, other medications, and blood glucose–monitoring supplies are temperature-sensitive, so avoid storing them in the trunk, glove compartment, back window of the car, or in a checked bag at the airport. Keep them in the original packaging so there's no question along the way as to what they are and who they belong to. And don't worry about the liquid carry-on limit on planes; the TSA allows you to exceed those limits for diabetes medications and supplies.

Tip #5: Carry snacks and treatment for low blood glucose. Food access is often unpredictable with travel, so carry portable snacks that won't spoil to head off hunger or treat low blood glucose (if you are at risk for that). See the previous list of "20 Travel-Friendly Foods." Also stash glucose tablets, gels, or hard candy in your pocket, carry-on bag, and wallet for easy access.

Tip #6: Have emergency contact and healthcare team contact information handy. Compiling this information in one place simplifies things if an emergency should arise and you need to get hold of them. Many people store this information in their wallet and/or on their smart phone.

Tip #7: Favor your feet. Wear well-fitting, comfortable shoes and socks at all times. Consider wearing light compression stockings if on a long flight or road trip, or if your feet swell otherwise. Check your feet frequently for blisters, cuts, or sores—especially after long walks.

Tip #8: Be prepared in the event you need medical care while traveling. Keep a small first aid kit handy. Before travel, check out local doctors in the area surrounding your destination who treat diabetes (and who speak English, if traveling abroad). Identify where local hospitals are. If you have access through your medical insurance to doctors online, set up your profile in the portal before you head out. Make sure you take your medical insurance card (and travel medical coverage if out of the country).

Tip #9: Keep a closer check on blood glucose. New foods, increased activity, and different time zones can throw your blood glucose off, so check more frequently, especially before and after meals.

Tip #10: The best defense is a good offense. First and foremost, when traveling, try to stay as close to your usual food and medication schedule as possible. Granted, that may be easier said than done, particularly when factoring in flight delays, road construction, traffic jams, and time-zone changes. If you take insulin and will be crossing time zones, talk with your healthcare team before your trip so they can help you plan the timing of your insulin injections and meals. Keep in mind that westward travel means a longer day (so possibly more insulin will be needed), and eastward travel means a shorter day (so possibly less insulin will be needed). By planning for the unexpected, you'll be ready when any travel-related eating or medication challenges come your way. After all, the best defense is a good offense.

10 Additional Travel Tips for Going Abroad

No one likes to think about the possibility of needing medical care while on a trip. However, advance planning can bring peace of mind when traveling outside the country and help you be prepared should a health event arise. Here are 10 tips to help you prepare for international travel (note, this is not an all-inclusive list):

1. Get appropriate immunizations.
2. One month before you leave, visit your healthcare team for a checkup.
3. Make plans for temporary health insurance coverage if your plan is not effective outside the U.S.
4. Write down a few diabetes-related phrases in the language of the country you're visiting, such as, "I have diabetes," "I need sugar," or "Where is the hospital?"

5. Wear diabetes identification in the languages of the countries you're visiting.
6. Use bottled water to drink and brush your teeth.
7. Avoid raw fruits and vegetables.
8. Skip beverages with ice.
9. Eat only dairy products that are pasteurized.
10. Always carry snacks with you.

Next Steps

1. List two eating strategies you can put into practice at your next family, holiday, or other social gathering.
2. If you drink alcohol, identify one nonalcoholic beverage that you could drink at your next event to help spread out and reduce alcohol consumption.
3. List two eating strategies or tips you will put into practice on your next trip.

Food for Thought

- Planning ahead and making intentional choices at social gatherings are essential to managing blood glucose and weight.
- If you choose to drink alcohol, practice moderation, with no more than one alcoholic drink per day if you are a woman and no more than two drinks per day if you are a man.
- When traveling, try to stay as close to your usual food and medication schedule as possible. And keep plenty of travel-friendly foods on hand.

LOOKING BACK, LOOKING AHEAD

CHAPTER 13

Eating Healthy with Diabetes Is a Journey, Not a Sprint

Y ou have reached the end of the book, and without a doubt, we have covered *a lot* of information. You've received some specific guidance on what to eat and learned about a variety of aspects of diabetes nutrition. My hope is that you feel you have the valuable information you need to make healthy choices. You may find you still have many things to think about and process. As mentioned in the Introduction, you need to prioritize what you want to accomplish and set goals. Overhauling every aspect of your eating habits could feel very overwhelming, but starting with changes that seem fairly easy to make may seem doable. Start with the low-hanging fruit, so to speak. Or start with changes where you'll get the most bang for your buck. Eating healthy is a journey. It is shaped by many factors, from the foods you like (and don't like), to where you are in life, and your traditions, culture, and personal choices over time. All of your food and beverage choices count.

What Stage of Change Are You In Now?

In the Introduction, we reviewed the stages of change. *In relation to healthy eating with diabetes, which stage were you in before you read this book?*

- Pre-contemplation?
- Contemplation?

- Preparation?
- Action?
- Maintenance?

Which stage do you find yourself in now?

Maybe you've been **contemplating** making change, and have now **prepared** for change, or taken **action** and are already making some changes.

Consider the Positive Things You're Doing, and Do More of Them

As you have learned, diabetes isn't like the majority of medical conditions. A simple pill or procedure won't just take care of it or make it go away. Although you do have the resources of your diabetes healthcare team, ultimately you are the one making the daily decisions that affect your health and well-being. As you learned in the Introduction, a general goal, such as "I want to lose weight," is not going to be easy to achieve unless you consider specific strategies that will work for you, such as "I'll get 30 minutes of exercise 5 days a week" or "I'll eat smaller portions at dinner each day." Setting specific, measurable, attainable, relevant, and timely goals (SMART goals) that work with your particular lifestyle will be easier for you to reach and will, in turn, give you the confidence you'll need to meet the challenges ahead.

Revisit the three SMART goals around healthy eating that you set and prioritized in the Introduction . . . *which have you already been able to accomplish? Or take steps toward*

accomplishing? How can you continue to do more of the positive things you're now already doing?

You deserve a huge congratulations on any positive changes you've been able to make! Small changes add up over time. The best plan is one that works for you to achieve your health goals, feel well, and live your best life. If you commit to doing the best you can do, then you've given it your all!

It's What You Do Most of the Time That Matters

Occasionally "life happens," and you may end up eating or drinking something that may send your blood glucose out of range or that may not be optimal for your health. No one is perfect. Rather than beating yourself up, take the opportunity to learn from the situation and plan what you could do differently next time.

Continue to Learn All You Can

A wise man once said, "Experience is a hard teacher. She gives the test first, and then the lesson afterward." The same thing applies to life with diabetes. You will find that you gain much by learning from each situation you face. *What worked when you were faced with a party buffet? How can you do that again next time? Or what will you do differently the next time you're traveling?*

With this book as your guide, through the "Next Steps" at the end of each chapter, you have accomplished the following specific tasks

---

Are You "Cheating" Yourself?

Have you ever felt guilty because you ate a cupcake, skipped a workout, or couldn't resist the lure of a late-night snack? People often use the word "cheat" to express the shame they feel after making a decision they wish they hadn't. If you find that you're beating yourself up with negative self-talk, here are three tips to keep in mind:

1. **The fact that you made an eating decision you wish you hadn't is not as important as what you're going to do about it now**. Don't let an unhealthy choice be an excuse to give up.
2. **Think about why you made the choice that you did.** *Were you feeling stressed? Did you let yourself get too hungry?* Learn from this situation and plan for what you'll do when you find yourself there again in the future. Next time, maybe you'll treat yourself to a stress-relieving walk or a funny sitcom instead of grabbing a chocolate bar.
3. **You're setting yourself up for failure if you expect perfection.** There will always be temptations, whether it's potato chips or pecan pie. Work with your registered dietitian nutritionist to figure out how to fit in special treats in a healthier way.

---

to set you on the path to eating well to manage diabetes:

- Reflected on changes you may have already made, what is going well, and identified how you can do more of that to continue down the path toward living your best life
- Assessed your physical activity and if you get enough
- Identified one swap you can make to cut calories
- Identified one way you can fit more movement or steps into your day
- Identified one tactic you can try to help manage stress
- Identified which eating pattern appeals to you and seems to be a good fit to help you achieve your goals
- Identified one change or swap you could make to begin embracing a new eating pattern
- Practiced portioning your plate following the Diabetes Plate Method
- Began compiling a list of favorite foods and carbohydrate counts of portions you frequently eat
- Evaluated what you drink and where there's opportunity to fit in more water

- Talked with your diabetes healthcare team about the best carbohydrate goal for you so you can get on your way with counting carbohydrate
- Rated your plate and how it aligned with the Diabetes Plate Method
- Kept a log for 3–4 days of everything that you eat and drink
- Took inventory of whether you could switch out some foods to improve your fat quality, trim sodium, and boost your fiber
- Checked the portion sizes of your meat servings
- Tried to fit in fish
- Put your label-reading skills to the test
- Put your measuring and weighing food and beverage skills to the test
- Planned three menus for the next week
- Selected one new shopping strategy to try
- Found one new recipe to try that fits your preferences and health goals
- Savored the joy of eating
- Practiced identifying foods at your favorite takeout or fast-food dining venues that fit the suggested carbohydrate goals for three meals
- Listed two swaps or changes that you can make to restaurant meals so they fit your diabetes eating plan
- Checked your blood glucose 1 1/2– 2 hours after eating out to see if it is in the target range for your blood glucose levels
- Listed three snacks you can eat at home that meet your taste and nutrition needs
- Listed three snacks you can eat on the go that meet your taste and nutrition needs
- Listed two strategies you can try to keep snacks and snack portions healthy
- Listed five favorite recipes that you could renew by making a few ingredient swaps and picked one to work on
- Listed two eating strategies you can put into practice at your next family, holiday, or other social gathering
- If you drink alcohol, identified one **nonalcoholic** beverage that you could drink at your next event to help spread out and reduce alcohol consumption
- Listed two eating strategies or tips you will put into practice on your next trip

Each of these accomplishments took you one step further along the path to healthy eating and managing diabetes. But the learning doesn't stop here! When you put down this book, you might be surprised to suddenly notice the vast amount of available information about diabetes and nutrition.

Some of the advice you receive about diabetes will be given by well-meaning family members and friends. Other information might come from the popular press or your own Internet searches. *How do you sort out the helpful advice from the old wives' tales? Fact from fiction?* Not everything you hear, read, or see is based on science or confirmed by research.

Internet Insight: Reliable Diabetes and Healthy-Eating Information

A seemingly endless amount of diabetes information is available on the Internet. The problem is figuring out whether this information is safe and reliable. Be skeptical. Things that sound too good to be true often are. **To find the best health resources, ask these four questions:**

1. Who sponsors the website you are browsing? Is it a reputable source? Look for an "About Us" page.
2. What are the credentials of those who provide information for the site? Does the site have an editorial board?
3. When was the site last updated? Health information is constantly changing.
4. What does your diabetes healthcare team think about the information you've found? Information you find on a website does not replace your healthcare team's advice.

One Experience with Unreliable Internet Information: "White Foods Are Bad"

Many times throughout my years in practice, I've had clients come in voicing the belief that "white foods are bad for diabetes," based on a story they read online.

The belief that people with diabetes should avoid all white foods is false. The idea of avoiding anything white seems to have blossomed out of the focus on reducing carbohydrate. The phrase "white foods are bad" is an oversimplification and a source of confusion. While originally the intent of this phrase was related to avoiding refined grains, many have taken it literally over the years and avoided good-for-you white foods that are part of a healthy eating pattern—such as low-fat milk or yogurt, white beans, onions, cauliflower, and bananas.

Takeaway: Just because you read information online or on social media does not mean it's true. Ask yourself the questions in the Internet Insight box above and talk it over with your healthcare team.

Websites with Valuable and Reliable Information About Diabetes and Healthy Eating

Diabetes

American Diabetes Association
www.diabetes.org

JDRF (formerly Juvenile Diabetes Research Foundation)
www.jdrf.org

National Diabetes Education Program (NDEP)
www.ndep.nih.gov

National Institutes of Health—MedlinePlus
www.nlm.nih.gov

Healthy Eating

Academy of Nutrition and Dietetics
www.eatright.org

ChooseMyPlate (USDA)
www.choosemyplate.gov

Diabetes Food Hub (American Diabetes Association)
www.diabetesfoodhub.org

Dietary Guidelines for Americans
www.health.gov/dietaryguidelines

U.S. Department of Agriculture (USDA) Food and Nutrition Information Center
http://fnic.nal.usda.gov

Build Your Personal Support Team

Having support navigating life with diabetes is equal in importance to getting education about diabetes to know how to manage it. People who have a strong support system in place tend to be healthier and recover more quickly when they are sick.

Support comes in many forms. Maybe it's someone to walk or exercise with to keep you accountable. Or someone to cook with. It could be someone to talk to about life's challenges and cheers you up or someone who's your encourager. Or it may be your diabetes care and education specialist, registered dietitian nutritionist, or diabetes healthcare team.

Reach Out to Your Diabetes Healthcare Team

If you have questions or concerns about diabetes, your eating plan, or other aspects of management, ask your diabetes healthcare team. They are dedicated to helping you take an active role in caring for your diabetes.

Reach Out to Family and Friends

Many of the healthy-eating principles you implement to manage diabetes are good for your family as well, making it easier for them to join you in support. Often, family and friends want to help but don't understand diabetes or know exactly how to offer help. They may seem more like the diabetes police than a diabetes ally. It may help for you to share specific ways they can support you (such as, "**Do** join me in making healthy lifestyle changes, but please **don't** offer unsolicited advice about my eating.")

Reach Out to Others with Diabetes

In time, you may be ready to widen your support network by joining a support group, participating in a diabetes program or workshop, or connecting with others in the vibrant online diabetes community. The American Diabetes Association has an online discussion board that allows people with diabetes to share their ideas, questions, and opinions on a variety of topics. These settings provide great opportunities to discuss common problems and concerns as well as share helpful advice, offer support, and celebrate success in diabetes self-care. Another great way to reach out is to participate in an organized activity that focuses on diabetes, such as a walk, bike ride, or health fair. Participating in these events is a fun way for you to make a difference in your local community by raising awareness or raising money for the research and treatment of diabetes. There is strength in numbers. You are not alone on your journey with diabetes!

I encourage you to consider what types of support could help you now. Where will you get it? And when will you take the step to see this support?

In Summary: The Nutrition Guidelines for Diabetes

Table 13.1 contains a summary of the general guidelines addressed throughout this book based on the latest science and research. To re-emphasize what I noted at the beginning of this book, I encourage you to meet with a registered dietitian nutritionist to develop an individualized meal plan based on your needs, goals, and personal food preferences.

TABLE 13.1	GUIDELINES YOU'VE LEARNED IN THIS BOOK
Nutrient	**Nutrition Guidelines for Diabetes**
Calories	You may need to reduce the number of calories you eat to lower your blood glucose and promote weight loss. Reducing just 500 calories from your daily intake could mean a weight loss of 1 pound each week.
Carbohydrate	The amount (grams) of carbohydrate and available insulin have a strong influence on the way your blood glucose reacts after you eat. Reducing your carbohydrate is a key strategy to improve blood glucose. See Chapter 4 for more details.

(continued)

TABLE 13.1	GUIDELINES YOU'VE LEARNED IN THIS BOOK (Continued)
Nutrient	**Nutrition Guidelines for Diabetes**
Fiber and whole grains	Your fiber and whole-grain goals should be the same amount recommended for the other members of your family: a minimum of 14 grams for every 1,000 calories consumed or about 25 grams of fiber each day for adult women and 38 grams of fiber each day for adult men. At least half of all the grains you eat should be whole grains. See Chapter 5 for more details.
Protein	If you have normal kidney function, your intake of protein foods (meats, poultry, seafood, dairy foods, beans, peas, nuts, and seeds) should be the same as that of the general public. That would cover about one-fourth of a 9-inch plate. See Chapters 3 and 5 for more details.
Fat	There is no proven ideal quantity of fat recommended for people with diabetes; however, quality or type of fat is important for heart health. Foods higher in unsaturated fats (liquid fats) are healthier than solid saturated and trans fats. See Chapter 5 for more details. A registered dietitian nutritionist can help you learn more about heart-healthy unsaturated fats and how to avoid saturated and trans fats, as well as identify the right amount of fat for you. Lower fat intake can also translate into lower calorie intake, which may help you maintain a reasonable body weight.
Vitamins, minerals, and herbal supplements	The American Diabetes Association does not recommend any special vitamins, minerals, or herbal supplements as a general rule for individuals with diabetes. Vitamin B12 levels should be monitored in individuals taking metformin.
Alcohol	If you choose to drink alcohol, use it in moderation: one drink or fewer per day if you're a woman or two drinks or fewer per day if you're a man. Alcohol may increase the risk of hypoglycemia. See Chapter 12 for more details.
Sodium	Sodium recommendations for people with diabetes are similar to recommendations for the general population: <2,300 milligrams per day. See Chapter 5 for more details.
Sweeteners	A number of zero-calorie and reduced-calorie sweeteners are approved for use in the U.S. People with diabetes are advised to limit or avoid sugar-sweetened beverages to reduce the risk of weight gain and cardiovascular disease. See Chapter 4 for more details.

Source: Evert AB, Dennison M, Gardner CD, et al. Nutrition Therapy for Adults with Diabetes or Prediabetes: A Consensus Report. *Diabetes Care* 2019;42:731–754.

In Closing

As you've learned through reading this book, there is no "one-size-fits-all" diet for managing diabetes. There are a variety of eating patterns, approaches, and tools. It's good to have options. Everyone is different. The end goal is finding what works for you to keep your blood glucose in range, and then doing more of that. My hope is that you feel like you have an answer to the question, "What do I eat now?", and that you are more confident about putting healthy eating into practice to help simplify life with diabetes and live your best life. Take it one meal, one day, and one week at a time. Small changes add up!

Next Steps

1. Think of a situation in which you have been tempted to overeat. Make a plan for what you'll do when you find yourself in a similar situation again.
2. List the positive changes you've made in your eating habits and lifestyle.
3. Continue working on the SMART goals you set in the Introduction. When these goals are achieved, set new ones to continue making progress and moving forward.

Food for Thought

- Healthy eating with diabetes is a journey, not a sprint.
- You are the manager of your eating pattern and lifestyle.
- Acknowledge the positive changes you've made and things you are doing. *How can you do more of it, more often?*
- Reach out to others for help and support.
- Continue to learn all you can about diabetes and healthy eating.

INDEX

Note: Page numbers followed by *t* refer to tables. Page numbers in **bold** refer to an in-depth discussion.